STANDARD SETTING
A Practical Approach

For Adrian

STANDARD SETTING

A Practical Approach

June Girvin

MACMILLAN

First published 1995 by
MACMILLAN PRESS LTD
Houndmills, Basingstoke, Hampshire RG21 2XS
and London
Companies and representatives
throughout the world

ISBN 0-333-59872-5

A catalogue record for this book is available
from the British Library.

10   9   8   7   6   5   4   3   2   1
04   03   02   01   00   99   98   97   96   95

Printed in Malaysia

Contents

Preface

I have wanted to write a book like this for a long time. Like a lot of first-time writers I thought that I did not have the skills required, and I could not quite believe that people would actually want to read what I might write. Kerry Lawrence, and later Margaret O'Gorman, both of the Macmillan Press, encouraged me to take the plunge and this text is the result. The book is based upon my experiences and expertise gained using the Royal College of Nursing's Dynamic Standard Setting System (DySSSy), and several years of working with nurses on monitoring and improving their practice.

DySSSy was developed into a usable framework by Professor Alison Kitson of the Royal College of Nursing's Dynamic Quality Improvement Programme based at the National Institute of Nursing, Oxford. I want to thank Alison for the support and practical assistance she has freely given me during the past five or six years and I unreservedly acknowledge her influence and her generosity. The founding members of the RCN's Quality Assurance Network (QUAN) have been a source of support and friendship over the years and have influenced my work and my career plans far more than I suspect they realise.

I also want to thank the nurses who contributed their stories and standards to this book and made the whole project possible, especially my clinical colleagues in Wales. If this book is a success it will be because of their candour and willingness to share not only their successes, but some of their more difficult moments too. Many of the comments quoted in the text were noted during workshops on standard setting and auditing carried out throughout Wales when the author was employed as Nursing and Midwifery Audit Co-ordinator (Wales) between 1991 and 1993. It was largely as a result of the comments and conversations from these workshops that the need for a simple text on standard setting became clear. I hope that this book goes some way towards meeting the needs of those nurses who welcomed me so enthusiastically into their work areas to help them with the mechanics of standard setting and monitoring.

Chrissy Dunn, Practice Development Nurse at Battle Hospital, Reading, has been an invaluable source of good sense and quiet advice. Without her to share the uncertainties, triumphs and tribulations of making quality assurance accessible and acceptable to busy nurses I would have given it all up long ago. Much of what is written here, Chrissy has been putting into practice for years. Long may she continue to do so.

I want to thank Poppy Moon, who made sense out of the figures for me, and Chris Baker who read and re-read numerous drafts of the text (until she could recite great chunks of it!) with enthusiasm and encouragement. Her staff of the Child and Adolescent Unit at the Royal Gwent Hospital, Newport, were some of the first nurses that I worked with using these techniques.

I acknowledge the assistance of Hazel Taylor, Director of Nursing and Quality, Glan Hafren NHS Trust (formerly South Gwent Health Unit) who gave permission for work undertaken when the author was employed there as Senior Nurse Special Projects between 1987 and 1991 to be used in some of the figures in this book.

Judith Potter and Ken Dolbear are to be thanked for allowing the use of a standard and audit tool resulting from a collaborative project between Social Services and the Swindon and Marlborough NHS Trust during the author's employment as Executive Director of Nursing and Quality.

Finally, I thank my husband, Adrian, who for the past nineteen years has believed in me totally and fiercely, and who must be heartily sick of eating, sleeping and breathing nursing and nursing developments! It is his contribution to my confidence that I am most grateful for.

June Girvin

Introduction

For much of the past six years I have been involved in standard setting with clinical nurses. When I first started out I did not have a clue – I did not know what a standard was, or how to go about writing one, or how it might be used. There were countless occasions when I wished that someone had written a simple text that might help me. Six years on, Macmillan have given me the opportunity to write that simple text myself, and that is exactly what I hope I have done – prepared a simple handbook on the mechanics of standard setting for those who want to have a go but are not sure of where to start.

Almost every day at work I meet with nurses who are confused about quality assurance activities – I hear complaints about remoteness and irrelevance to practice, and there is an unsurprising reluctance to get involved in activities that are meaningless. I meet with other nurses who have a genuine desire to get to grips with standards but who have been totally confused by inadequate training, conflicting methods, and the all too common problem of the organisation flitting from one quick fix for quality to another.

In the areas of England and Wales where I have been actively and persistently involved with nurses setting standards, I have seen the changes, improvements and motivation that such an approach can encourage. When people know what they are doing, standard setting is a wonderful mechanism for making things happen. It works. Knowing what you are doing, however, takes a bit of practice, and requires encouragement, coaching, a good grasp of the practical skills and knowledge of where those practical skills fit into the bigger picture. Standards are part of a whole cycle of activities – identifying areas for improvement, setting the standard that you want to reach, monitoring that standard, and taking any remedial action required. These component parts cannot be separated – must not be separated. Standards are pointless if you are not going to attempt to improve upon them, pointless if you are not going to monitor them, pointless if you have no intention of acting upon the results of your monitoring.

Standard setting is only one link in a chain of activities – it is a means to an end and **never** an end in itself. It is the first step into practical quality improvement. It is not just fine words and clever theories, but a truly practical way of tackling quality improvement in a busy work environment.

The aim of this book is to provide nurses (primarily, though I hope the book will be useful for others) with limited experience of standard setting with an introduction to the basic skills required and some down to earth advice on how to get started and keep going through the whole chain of activity. It is not an academic reader on quality assurance, but a simple handbook of techniques. It has its limitations, and I freely acknowledge them – some will accuse me of being simplistic, of not giving enough background information, of not setting the subject in context, of being mechanistic, and so on. Some may decry its informal style or its amateur approach.

I have written this book in the same way that I speak, and I have relied upon my editor to let me know when this does not work. I have run successful workshops and have given some well-received talks and papers on standard setting – I hope the style is equally successful in print.

The quality of nursing care provided to patients is very important to me. Important enough to have led me to take a number of jobs through which I have tried to influence a wider and wider section of the profession. Equally important to me is finding ways of helping nurses to understand how they can make the quality of their care explicit, how they might monitor that quality and how they can influence what happens in their sphere of practice through standards. I hope that those who read and use this book will find themselves beginning to appreciate how standard setting can be an educational device, a mechanism for change, an organisational tool and a springboard for professional development. Yes, it can be all of these things.

All of my experience in working with standards has been gained using the Royal College of Nursing's Dynamic Standard Setting System (DySSSy). I have worked with the RCN's Standards of Care team, now the Dynamic Quality Improvement team, since I started in standards and much of what I have learned has come through them. This book uses the basic principles of DySSSy throughout, and all the examples follow its format to a lesser or greater degree. However, this book is about how I use DySSSy and as such may differ occasionally from the original. DySSSy is an excellent framework, but you have to make it work through people; you have to understand its mechanics and you have to realise its philosophy. Any standards contained in this text are not meant to be seen as good or bad examples. They are simply there to illustrate the relevant point, and should not be seen as cast in tablets of stone or examples of excellence. I am sure that they will be scrutinised and judged by anyone who has ever written a standard – it is important to remember that they have been written by nurses (and occasionally other professionals) at varying stages of development and with varying levels of expertise. They are examples based on actual practice experiences and were not written especially for this book, but were freely given to be used as illustrations.

The aim of this book is to give more nurses the confidence to participate in and influence the quality and audit processes in their workplace. If this is achieved it will have been well worth the effort of the last eighteen months.

CHAPTER 1

Where to Start

We were told to have six standards written and ready by the end of the month. No one had any idea of what to do and there was no help offered – just an expectation that we would produce these standards at the end of the month and that would be that.

Ward Sister, District General Hospital

I hear this kind of thing so often and it always makes me angry and frustrated. Do you remember when the 'nursing process' was introduced – overnight, practically – and how nobody knew what they were supposed to be doing and how it became a paper exercise in so many places? Exactly the same mistakes have been made and are still being made with standard setting. No preparation, no education, no support – and then people wonder why it does not seem to be doing what it is supposed to do.

When you are working in difficult and almost impossibly busy situations you do not need directives to do even more work without any support and assistance. Particularly if you cannot see any reason for doing it, and particularly if it does not seem to be terribly relevant to you. Right at the outset you need to understand why you should spend time on standard setting and what might be the possible benefits.

Everyone knows what their own standards are – they are inside us and act as an unconscious guide to our practice. The problem is, we may not all have the same standards – one nurse's excellence may be another nurse's idea of near negligence. Some nurses know more than others, some work harder, some try harder, some are interested in what they are doing and some are not. All in all it can lead to inconsistency in practice. You might want to consider how reasonable it is for patients to receive good care on one shift and not such good care on the next, or good care when a particular nurse is looking after them and not such good care when it is someone else. Should patients not expect a consistent standard of care no matter who is caring for them?

It is very hard for us all to give the same level of care to patients if that level of care, that is, the *standard*, has not been made explicit and agreed between all nurses in the team. You cannot give a good standard of care if you are not sure what a good standard is. And if you are inexperienced, or you have not had opportunities to update yourself, then you may well be unsure about what 'good care' is in a given situation. A written standard is one way of letting everyone know what the level of care that you want to give is. It states specifically and openly what you expect to happen.

So, already we have two good reasons for thinking about spending time on standards: we have an obligation to provide consistency to the people who put their trust in us; and by sharing our ideas on good care with each other we can get an agreement on the level of care that we want everyone to provide in our particular work area – we can make our expectations clear to each other.

There are also strong political reasons for having some sort of written standards. Clear, written standards can be useful in any discussions you may have with managers about your role and the work you carry out. Nursing is notoriously difficult to define, and I am not suggesting for one minute that a few standards will do what a lifetime's debate is still struggling with, but they will help you to demonstrate to your managers how your ward operates, how you operationalise your values and how you endeavour to meet patients' needs If your manager can actually *see* what you are trying to achieve, and can easily identify the implications of not meeting a part of the standard, it may well improve your communication and should at least improve their understanding of your objectives.

Sometimes care is affected by factors other than our own expertise or knowledge. There are environmental factors which affect care, or activities performed by other health carers that impact upon the care that we, as nurses, can give. You can probably reel off a whole list of these, and on the top of that list, I am quite sure, will be staffing levels, closely followed by other resource deficiencies, and inefficiencies of the system, and so on.

When you start to set standards, you have to think about these things too. You have to consider the environment that you work in and the facilities and resources that are available to you. You have to make decisions about what you can, and what you cannot, reasonably do. You have to think about spheres of control, and who can make things happen. For example, a group of nurses on a continuing care ward wanted to improve their patients' meals. They identified the main problems as being the following:

● huge portions and subsequent waste
● continental dishes which their patients would not eat
● vegetables which were not cooked soft enough.

Fired with enthusiasm, the group started to write a standard which specified the changes required. It was well into their second meeting when realisation dawned that although they could identify these problems, the solutions

3

to them were not in their sphere of control. Unless the catering department got involved, nothing at all was likely to happen. So, a whole round of new negotiations had to start – inviting the catering manager to join the group, discussing the issues sensitively (**not** presenting the man with a list of his department's shortcomings and expecting him to do as he was told!) and agreeing possible goals and changes to be made. At the end of the day it turned out to be a very successful standard (see the Further Reading section at the back for a fuller account) and is a good example of how multidisciplinary audit might get off the ground.

Try to make sure that you have got the right people together to make your standard work, and make sure that you are looking at a topic that you can actually do something about. Choosing a subject for standard setting can be difficult – especially if you are new to it and you have been 'presented' with a list of topics to set standards on by someone else.

One good way of starting is to view standard setting as a means of tackling problems. In the example of the meals service, the nurses identified one aspect of care on their ward that they were not happy about – in this case it was the meals service, but it could just as easily have been the incidence of pressure sores, the way that patients were admitted, discharge planning arrangements, safety in the play room – any number of things. If you choose to look at areas that you know are unsatisfactory, then the chances are that you will achieve some improvement; you will get a sense of what success with standards can be like, and you may well be motivated to go on and work on another topic. Problem solving with standards is a good way to start – you get results while you are learning.

Standard setting is not only useful for problem solving, it can also be used for other purposes. It may well be that your ward is actually very effective in a certain

4

aspect of care – perhaps you have excellent discharge planning arrangements which work brilliantly, perhaps you have worked out a way of preparing patients psychologically for theatre which seems to help them. Other wards may not be so successful and it may be a case of 'What do they do that we don't?' and 'Why do they get so few post-discharge problems?' In this sort of situation a standard which reflects your good practice may be useful for other wards and departments, so that they can learn from you, and perhaps even adapt your standard to their own work area. This sharing of work is an exciting part of standard setting and is often a way of moving towards broader standards for a clinical unit – you retain the individual relevance for your own ward, but there is some recognition of core criteria appearing in all standards written on a particular theme. (Perhaps with work and refinement these are the essential elements that could be offered into the contracting process? If so then this could be the start of practice really beginning to influence policy making. Small beginnings – but with that vision in front of you, it's not as impossible as you might think!)

You probably already realise that you have to have everyone on board in standard setting, and you also probably know that a good way of getting commitment to a project is to get people involved in it. *Ownership* is a key word in standard setting and it really is crucial. There are probably quite a lot of people reading this book who know of a nice fat file of standards on the office shelf at work, written by a manager or a quality specialist, and handed out to the ward for you to follow. Do you follow them? Do you ever! My guess is, you had a look through them, decided that they were all very well but there were bits that were not relevant to your ward, parts of standards that were way out of line, things that you could never achieve even if you spent the rest of your life working on them. You probably rolled your eyes, and stuck the file on the shelf, where it has stayed ever since.

And it does not really matter, because nobody has mentioned them since they appeared, and there are no attempts to measure them. 'Standards? Oh, yes, we've done that, they don't work.' And that is quite right – irrelevant, imposed, and impossible standards do not work. But if standards are about issues that are important to your ward team, if they address your particular care priorities, if they are relevant to your ward and your staff, and take into account your environment and facilities and resources and do not set unachievable targets – might you feel differently about them then? If you had been involved in writing them, in deciding what went in them, and what could be left out, deciding on a level of care that you could achieve and that you would feel confident about monitoring because you had a say in what was written down – might you be feeling differently? If you had decided what the standards needed to be about, if you could address certain problems with them, use them to focus on areas of concern, write standards that meant something to you in practical terms rather than something plucked out of the air simply to complete the paper exercise – wouldn't you be more interested then? Of course you would. And so would practically everyone else on your ward or in your area of work. Motivation to do something means that you are halfway to getting it finished. One of the strongest motivators of all is personal commitment. You have to want to do it for your own reasons. Not because it is flavour of the month, not because you do not have any choice, not because it is a social or a professional obligation, but because you *want* to do it. Those other things all help but you have to want to work at making things better in your own work area.

Unfortunately, the fact that you are committed to doing something is not enough in itself. You cannot write standards if you do not know how to. Find someone who has some experience of standards and get them to help you. Better still, get someone in your place of work trained as a standards facilitator and then they can help everyone. It is difficult to teach yourself, but it is not impossible. This book, I hope, will go some way towards helping you to start standard setting and there are other publications that you will also find helpful (see Further Reading, pp. 103–4).

You cannot write standards on your own – if they are meant to reflect the standards of your ward, then the whole nursing team (or wider professional team, depending upon the standard) needs to be involved. As I wrote earlier, your standards may be quite different from someone else's, but what you are looking for is a standard for everyone to work to – that means a standard that everyone agrees with and thinks is reasonable. The easiest way to get agreement is to make sure that everyone contributes to the standard. Practically, this is a very difficult thing to do in busy clinical areas. It is not realistic to expect all the nurses on a ward or within a department to get together with a facilitator to talk standards every Friday afternoon for a couple of hours. One way around this problem is to identify a couple of people who are able to meet regularly with the facilitator within their clinical setting, and then everyone else drops into meetings as and when they can be spared. One person from the regular group is responsible for making sure that anything agreed at the meeting is drafted out and that every nurse on the ward sees it (including night staff and part-timers), comments on it, and adds anything or takes out anything that they feel strongly about. This amended draft standard comes back to the regular group and is checked through and agreed, and then it goes out again, and so on, until a final draft is ready that everyone on the ward is happy with. It takes a little while but it is a realistic way of involving everyone, and it does mean that you are more likely to get ownership and a much greater chance of real commitment to making the standard work.

Having mentioned that a facilitator may help you with the work, it is important that you have a good idea of what a facilitator is and what their role entails. There can be a lot of misconceptions concerning facilitators. For example, some people think that anyone can be a facilitator. This is not really true. You need certain skills, and these can be learned, but I believe that you also need to have a certain sort of personality and you cannot necessarily learn that.

I have met quite a few people who have been 'given' the job of facilitator and some of them have been inappropriate choices, for lots of reasons. This is a personal view, but I have seen real problems caused by the following ideas:

● *If your job title contains the words 'quality assurance' or 'audit' then you are automatically a facilitator.*

This is a bit like saying that if you can talk to people you are a counsellor.

● *All nurse managers can be standards facilitators because it is the most convenient and cheap way of doing things.*

Occasionally, the last person a group of nurses want to discuss their practice with is their manager. Some will have the right level of credibility and acceptance, others will not.

● *You do not need to know anything about standard setting to be a standards facilitator – if you have facilitation skills, you can facilitate anything.*

This sounds reasonable, but I do not think it works. For example, I have a driving licence but I daresay I would need the odd lesson if I wanted to drive a 36 ton lorry. If the standard-setting group already has the practical skills then someone with good facilitation skills will be useful to them. If the standard-setting group are starting from scratch, as so many of them are in my experience, then the facilitator must have knowledge of the skills and techniques of standard setting.

You are probably already aware that not everyone means the same thing when they say 'facilitator'. It varies from a 'helper' to a 'chairman' to a 'group leader', with plenty of permutations between. This is what some nurses have said to me about facilitation and the need for it:

It's useful to have someone from outside of the ward area helping you, sometimes it's hard to see the wood for the trees yourself.

Enrolled nurse, Care of the Elderly ward

We would never have kept at it in the early days without our facilitator, it was such hard work. She kept us motivated and made sure that we understood what we were doing. It meant that later on she could withdraw without us giving up – we knew what to do and enjoyed doing it – we just called her in if there was something we couldn't work through ourselves, or if we weren't sure about anything.

Ward Sister, District General Hospital

When we first started we used to argue like mad over what should go in the standard and what shouldn't. Our facilitator took a lot of stick and soaked up quite a bit of that hostility so that it didn't break up the group. When you're not used to having your authority challenged it can be quite intimidating to find that your ward team don't actually automatically agree with your idea of a standard! The facilitator helped us to be

9

constructive and sort of 'depersonalised' the arguments for us.

Ward Sister, DGH

You can see just from these quotes that the facilitator needs to be quite sensitive, and certainly needs to be able to read a situation as it is unfolding. The facilitator has to assess

- when people need to be directed, and when it is better to leave them to get on with things in their own way;
- when to stop them making mistakes and when to let them experience the odd problem or two;
- when to stop actively helping and start supporting;
- how to get people back on track when they are getting carried away without cutting off their enthusiasm or making them feel as if they do not know anything.

It is a skilful role and a very privileged position to be in, and no one should just launch into it without some training or realisation of the responsibility that it carries.

At this point it might be worth considering one of the most common questions asked, and one of the most common mistakes made. The confusion between standards and procedures, and what the difference is between the two.

I see a lot of standards that are really just procedures – the procedure manual has simply been rewritten in a 'standard' type format, using structure, process, outcome or similar headings. You need to think very carefully about this – standards are about stating the level of care that has been agreed as desirable. It should cover much more than the specific actions required to carry out a task. This is actually quite difficult to explain and I think it is probably one of those things that suddenly dawn on you as your knowledge about standard setting increases. As you read on, and consider some of the examples, I hope that you will begin to appreciate for yourself how standards and procedures differ.

If you need a simple checklist to remind you how to carry out an isolated task that you are unsure about – you need a procedure. It reminds you of the equipment, and broadly how to go about the task in terms of physical actions. You might, for instance, need a procedure to remind you how to prepare certain drugs for intravenous administration. However, you may be concerned that nurses do not really understand the implications of giving certain drugs in this way, that they have never been properly educated and that though their mechanical technique may be sound, their background knowledge may make them unsafe in other ways, and it may mean that the patient is not being properly informed, and so on. In this case, a simple procedure is not enough and you need a *standard* which can address all of these issues in one go. You might consider a standard statement something like:

Patients prescribed IV drugs receive them safely and competently and have an awareness of the reasons for this method of administration being used.

Under this heading you can think about nurse education; restricting administration to particular nurses meeting certain criteria; how to explain drug regimes to the patient; what to do if you consider the route to be inappropriate; what you mean by safe and competent, and so on. This is much, much more than you would find in a procedure.

Standards should be about the level of care every patient can expect no matter what his or her condition or problems. The standard should apply to everyone identified by you as being an appropriate client group. The patients' individual needs will be met by their care plans,

11

and that will differ from patient to patient. However, the overall standard will apply to everyone.

As I said before, it is quite hard to explain it at this stage, but you will start to see the difference as we proceed.

So, at the end of this first chapter you will understand why you need the following things to get started on setting standards:

- To get a group together
- To have the right people in the group
- To have access to someone who can help you in the early stages
- To have some idea of what you need to write your standard about.

You also need to be prepared to make mistakes and for it to take time. Some of the groups I have worked with took as long as *four months* to get their first standard written, starting from scratch, with no previous experience or knowledge of standard setting, but with access to a facilitator. Please do not all close this book and give up straight away. All of those groups, once they had cut their teeth on one standard, wrote the second one much more quickly. I can say with confidence, that once you have written one or two standards, and you know what the pitfalls are, then you will be able to write them in the space of two or three meetings with no trouble at all. So, take heart, it really does get much easier with experience.

CHAPTER 2

Getting to Grips with SPO

This chapter will work through the mechanics of getting a standard down on paper. I will use the Royal College of Nursing's DySSSy format, because this is the approach with which I am most familiar and experienced. I also feel that it is easy to use once you have learned your way around it.

Many nurses use this type of format for their standard setting – identifying *Structures, Processes* and *Outcomes* – and I am sure that many of you will be familiar with these terms, or will at least have come across them. For the sake of clarity, I am going to explain each of these terms in the context of standard setting. It is important to remember that these definitions apply *within the context of standard setting* – the words structure, process and outcome can have other meanings outside standard setting and though it can be confusing, we have to learn to live with differing interpretations. Once you understand how the interpretation of these words is reliant upon the context then you will also avoid getting into unnecessary arguments about the meaning of words.

In Chapter 1 we talked about a standard being an agreed level of care that we wanted everyone in our area to work to. A standard statement is a sentence which briefly reflects the purpose of the standard, for example;

Patients with diabetes are able to estimate their own blood sugar competently

or:

All patients receive pressure area care which reflects their at risk status

These statements are fine – as far as they go. They tell us about a result – what we want to see happening; but they do not tell us how to make it happen. They do not tell us what we might need, or what to do. This is where the rest of the standard comes in. We need to develop some *criteria* which tell us how to make the standard statement happen.

These criteria make up the three columns in the standard and they consist of structure criteria, process criteria and outcome criteria.

Working out which criteria is which took us quite a while. Before it was properly explained to us we thought you could put anything anywhere!

Staff Nurse, Paediatric Unit

At first I got really confused over structure and process criteria, just a change in tense or the way you constructed the sentence made such a difference. It would have been easy to give up at this point – it just seemed too complicated.

Health Visitor

Structure criteria tell us what we need to have in place in order to make the standard happen. If our expectation is that diabetic patients are going to be able to measure their own blood sugar competently, what do we need to have in place? We need someone to teach them the required practical skills, we need equipment for them to use, we may need a policy or procedure to refer to, we need time to spend with the patient for teaching purposes. These things – staff, resources, equipment, documentation, and so on – these are all structures. *They are the things we need to have in place before the standard can happen.*

Process criteria tell us what activities we need to undertake in order to make the standard happen. Consider the diabetic patients again. If they are going to be able to monitor their own blood sugar competently, what do we have to do? We have to show the patients what to do carefully and slowly and explain exactly what they are required to do, we have to watch the patients and assess their competence, we have to decide on an alternative strategy if any patients cannot manage to do it for themselves, we have to document our findings so that colleagues are aware of the patients' progress. These things – things that the nurse does, explains, ensures, and so on, or that the patient does, are all processes. *They tell us the things that have to be done in order to make the standard happen.*

Then there are the *outcome criteria*. How do we know if the standard is happening? How do we know if our diabetic patients are able to monitor their own blood sugar competently? What are the things that will tell us if this is happening? The patients will be able to tell us what equipment they need and if they need to keep it anywhere special, they will be able to demonstrate the monitoring technique to us, they will be able to tell us what they will do if the result is too high or too low. These criteria will help us to judge their competence. They are called outcomes. *They are the outcomes for this particular standard* (see Figure 2.1 for full standard).

Be warned – in health care outcomes come in all shapes and sizes and in all sorts of disguises. Some people will tell you that these are not real outcomes, because they are not the result of a form of treatment. Some might say

15

Figure 2.1
Standard Setting Text

Standard Reference No:
Topic:
Care Group:
Achieve Standard by:
Review Standard by:

This standard is applicable in the
following wards/depts/areas:

Signature:
Signature:
Date:

STANDARD STATEMENT: DIABETIC PATIENTS ARE ABLE TO MEASURE THEIR OWN BLOOD SUGAR COMPETENTLY		
STRUCTURE	PROCESS	OUTCOME
S1 Nursing staff have knowledge of the importance of accurate blood sugar estimation in diabetes mellitus.	P1 A nurse issues the booklet to the patient prior to instructing him/her on how to monitor his/her own blood sugar.	01 Diabetic patients are able to demonstrate competently to the nurse how to estimate their own blood sugar as accurately as possible.
S2 Nursing staff have knowledge of the normal and abnormal range of blood sugar levels.	P2 A qualified nurse teaches the patient how to estimate his/her own blood sugar, demonstrating the technique carefully and as often as required.	02 Diabetic patients can state why it is important to record their blood sugar estimation.
Appropriate documentation is available:	P3 The qualified nurse assesses the patient's competence in monitoring his/her own blood sugar before discharge and records this in the nursing documentation.	03 Diabetic patients can tell the nurse what the normal/ abnormal blood sugar ranges are, and can state the action they would take if their own levels fall out of the normal range.
S3 A supply of blood glucose booklets is available. A supply of monitoring diaries is available.	P4 The nurse issues a diary to the patient and teaches him/her how to record blood sugar results in the diary, explaining the importance of keeping an accurate record.	
S4 Time is set aside for nurses to teach patients how to estimate their own blood sugar level.	P5 The nurse explains normal and abnormal blood sugar ranges, and advises the patient on action to take should their blood sugar fall out of the normal range.	
S5 A procedure on estimation of blood glucose levels is available on the ward.		

16

that they are not true outcomes but rather they are process outcomes. Fine, I am not going to get into an argument over meaning. For our purposes, and in the context
of this method of standard setting, they are outcomes. If
you are challenged over the use of this kind of statement
as an outcome, just explain that in the context of this
particular standard-setting method, yes, these qualify as
outcomes. That may not be what others are thinking of
when they talk of outcomes, but in this context, it is
acceptable.

Writing criteria seems easy, but takes a bit of getting
used to. Quite often you know what you want to say,
but it does not end up on the paper in quite the right
way. Staying with the diabetic education standard, it is
important that nurses use the appropriate documentation
when recording patients' progress, but you might end
up in a dilemma. For example – is it a structure?:

Appropriate documentation is available on the ward.

or is it a process?:

Nurses use appropriate documentation.

Or is it both? Well, think about it. Where is the best place
to put it? Appropriate documentation is obviously something that we have to have before we start, so it feels as
if it ought to be a structure. But, we also need to use
appropriate documentation, so it could reasonably be a
process. My advice would be to put it in the structure
column. Documentation is one of our resource/equipment
items, its place is in the structure column. I think that it
is safe to assume that if we have gone to the trouble of
specifically identifying a resource/piece of equipment, then
we expect it to be used. Putting it in the process column
would be superfluous and repetitive. The subsequent use
of the documentation is implicit. I hope that this shows

17

you how a small change in wording when you are constructing those criteria can change them very quickly from one sort to another. You have to know what you mean by structure, process and outcome; and you have to get that sentence just right so that it reflects exactly what you mean.

Usually, the structures, processes and outcomes are set down across the page in three columns. The commonest format is a landscape A4 (a large sheet of paper on its side), with the administrative details at the top; the standard statement set out clearly almost like a heading, and then three columns side by side for structure, process and outcome (see Figure 2.1 again). This is the format that the DySSSy system uses, and it is the format that I have always used and taught. Some people prefer to format their standards on a portrait A4 (using the piece of paper the 'right' way up). The administrative bit still comes at the top, the standard statement still forms a kind of header, but structure, process and outcome are set out one below the other. I do not think it really matters which way you choose to set out your standards, it is really just a matter of personal preference. As long as you understand the *principles* behind structure, process and outcome then the layout of your piece of paper is entirely up to you.

There are advantages and disadvantages to both landscape and portrait format and you should consider them before you make your choice, but really, whatever you are most comfortable using is probably best.

One of the first things I usually advise people in standard setting workshops is that your standards need to be short and concise. One page is plenty – more than one page and no one will bother to read them, it will be too much trouble. Standards have to be usable, every-day documents, so the less paper the better. The landscape format usually means that you can get your whole standard on one side of A4. You can see everything at a glance, and it is very convenient. Sometimes, because of this format, people confuse it with nursing process documentation and go into problem, plan and evaluation instead of structure, process and outcome and miss the point completely. A second problem that I come across frequently with this format is the tendency to make each criterion relate to the one in the column immediately to its left – thinking that the criteria have to read across the page and have to be linked together. This can create confusion and standards written like this usually contain a great deal of repetition and are often increasingly meaningless. For example, suppose we are writing a standard about reducing the risk of pressure damage. The first structure criterion is:

Nurses have a knowledge of causes and methods of prevention of pressure damage.

Fine. Then, we write a process to go with that structure that says:

Nurses receive regular, updated education on pressure damage prevention.

Then comes an outcome to follow which says:

Nurses have a knowledge of causes and methods of prevention of pressure damage.

Do you see the problem? The structure and the outcome are the same, and all three criteria seem to be saying the same thing only in slightly different words. Personally I really dislike this way of writing standards. I think it is unnecessary and you end up with a lot of nonsense in your standard. It is no wonder that people get put off!

Think hard about the standard statement, and how we have described the meaning of structure, process and outcome. If our aim is to reduce the incidence of pressure

19

damage then one of the things that we have to have, is nurses who *know* about pressure damage, otherwise the incidence of pressure damage cannot be reduced as no one knows how to achieve this. Knowledgeable nurses are a prerequisite for this standard. If we do not have knowledgeable nurses then our standard needs to be about education of staff rather than prevention of pressure damage. But, you might argue, when you write this standard you know that there are some nurses who do not know as much as they should and education needs to be a part of it. If this is the case, then put it in the structure. Put in something which says:

There is regular update training on prevention of pressure damage provided for all staff.

Or, try to see education as coming before the structures start, so that it becomes part of the implementation period before the standard is fully implemented. Another perspective is to exclude education because you expect nurses to possess this knowledge if the standard is to be achieved. However, on monitoring the standard you find that some nurses do not know enough. Education in this situation may become part of your action plan to get closer to the standard. Action plans will be covered later in the book, but I am just illustrating a point here. Confusing? It can be if you have never really thought about standard writing like this before. The whole point of this book is to help you think about your standard setting, so that even though it is a mechanism, you do not use it mechanistically, but you think about what you are putting where. You ensure that what goes down on the paper is exactly what you mean and cannot be misinterpreted. If not enough thinking and understanding goes on, then standard setting so often turns out to be a paper exercise.

When we first started we used the standards like the

nursing process – we thought that every structure had to have a matching process and outcome, like goals, plans and evaluations. Our standards were pages and pages long and we were worried that we would never really use them in practice.

Staff Nurse, Paediatric Unit

Try to think of your structure, process, and outcome criteria in lists. First, think of a list of all the things that you need to have (structures) in order to make the standard happen and write them down, then think of a list of all the things that you need to do (processes) in order to make the standard happen, then think of a list of all the things that will tell you if you have been successful (outcomes). Some of these will link with each other automatically – look for the links in the example in Figure 2.1. I am *not* saying that there must not be a link between structure, process and outcome, as that link is important if we are interested in outcome research. Also you will find that natural links are evident. What I *am* saying is do not force a link to be there – if there is not a natural link, then you could end up with repetitive 'baby talk'.

On to 'portrait' formatting. If you use a vertical page format (portrait) it can help you to avoid the last problem, because there is not the visual encouragement to move across the columns, but you also lose the visual sense of the standard as a whole. Using a vertical format means that it will be much more difficult to fit one standard on to one piece of paper – almost impossible I would say. As you will recall, more than one piece of paper may cause problems at a working level. How realistic is it to expect people to refer to two or even three sheets of paper, just to get the gist of an expectation of care? So, you will need to think carefully about your formatting. Once you know what you are doing, then you should not get the problems of 'baby talk' links; and once you have mastered the list approach then the visual and logistical benefits of a horizontal, (landscape) format become much more attractive.

Having read this far, you should be able to have a go at writing a standard for yourself. Do not expect it to be easy. It will take you a little while to get used to thinking about what you do in this way, and also to transferring those thoughts on to paper so that they are reasonable, sensible and easily understood by everyone.

Once you have sorted out your structures from your processes and your outcomes it is quite likely that you will have three lists that you have really just brainstormed. You might have some sentences, but you may also just have words – particularly under your structure list. For example, the pressure damage standard in Figure 2.2 might have looked something like this after an initial brainstorming session:

Structures

— Nurses' knowledge
— At risk scale
— Equipment, etc.
— Documentation

Processes

— Assessment of risk status – timescales
— Collaboration in plan with patient if possible
— Appropriate aids
— Evaluation and changes – who is responsible
— Patient education

Outcomes

— Less pressure damage or no pressure damage
— Care which reflects at risk status

Figure 2.2
Standard Setting Text

STANDARD STATEMENT: EVERY PATIENT RECEIVES PRESSURE AREA CARE APPROPRIATE TO THEIR NEEDS		
STRUCTURE	PROCESS	OUTCOME
S1 A trained nurse is available within 24 hours of admission to assess and plan patient's care.	P1 A trained nurse plans care with the collaboration of the patient and his or her relatives where this is possible.	01 Tissue damage is avoided by appropriate care, and incidence of pressure sores is reduced by x per cent.
S2 Every nurse has a knowledge of the causes and methods of prevention of pressure damage.	P2 Care is carried out as per the care plan and adjusted in the light of subsequent evaluation.	02 Patients receive preventative care according to their assessed needs.
S3 Nurses are aware of the policy on prevention of pressure sores.	P3 A risk indicator is used on admission and reassessed weekly on acute wards, monthly in long stay areas.	
S4 Lifting and Handling training is available to nurses.		
S5 A reliable risk indicator is in use.	P4 Lifting and movement of patients is carried out safely.	
S6 All nurses have a knowledge of the range of nursing aids available.	P5 Nurses ensure that appropriate preventative aids are used.	

You can see already that the number of criteria in each section is different – we have six structures, five processes and two outcomes. This is perfectly OK. Sometimes you might only have one outcome, and that might seem practically the same as the standard statement. That is OK as well. I have worked with a lot of nurses who worry if they only have one or two outcomes. They think that there must be something wrong, or that they must have missed something out. Often they will put in 'little extras' just to make more than one outcome. If the main purpose of your standard is to reduce the incidence of pressure damage, then one outcome which states that

23

pressure damage is reduced by x per cent is all that you need. Sometimes you may have secondary outcomes, it just depends on what you want your standard to achieve. Do not force things, and do not write things down just for the sake of it – think hard about exactly what you are aiming for.

Now you have to begin to turn this 'shorthand' into sentences which will make up your criteria. Remember that your standard needs to be concise if it is going to fit on one piece of paper, so every criterion must be strictly relevant to the standard statement. If your standard statement is about teaching diabetic patients to monitor their own blood sugar, then do not start writing criteria about testing their own urine. It is relevant in the total care, but for this particular standard it is irrelevant. Do not allow yourself to be side-tracked by related, but not strictly relevant issues.

Your criteria must also be measurable. This is an essential attribute. If you cannot measure it, then do not put it in your standard. Making your criteria measurable is not as difficult as it sounds – again it is often just about the way you construct your sentences. For example, think of the structure criterion from the earlier brainstorm of 'documentation'. You might think that it would be alright just to state 'documentation' in your structure column – after all, documentation is documentation, isn't it? But what is it about the documentation? What do you want to know about it?

You want to know that it is suitable for its purpose (that the correct documentation is being used), and that there is actually some documentation available for use. So, your structure criterion for documentation might say something like:

Appropriate documentation is available on the ward.

This tells you that you are looking for documentation

24

for use with patients who are being assessed for risk of developing pressure damage, and that you expect there to be a stock of it on the ward. Now this might seem a bit over the top, but when you come to monitor the standard, you will be grateful that you spelled it out in such detail.

You must also consider the achievability of your standard and its individual criteria. Standards and criteria must be achievable. What is the point in writing a standard that you know you cannot hope to reach? Why bother to monitor an unrealistic standard? – you know before you start that you are not going to meet it. You will need to consider achievability very carefully in discussion with your group. This does not mean that your standard has to be rock bottom – it does not preclude you from having to try a bit to meet it. But, it is important to be realistic and consider what you have available and the constraints that you work with. What can you reasonably expect to achieve?

Take the outcome for the pressure damage standard: should you go for an outcome of no incidence of pressure damage, or should you go for a percentage decrease on current incidence? This will depend on how much damage you currently have and the reasons for this. If, for example, your incidence is something like 25 per cent, then it may well be unrealistic to expect to drop it to zero in one swoop. It may be more sensible to state that it will be reduced to 10 per cent within three months, or by the time you monitor the standard next. When you do monitor, and if you have reduced it to 10 per cent, you can then review your criteria and think about changing your outcome again to perhaps 5 per cent incidence. In this way you can make bigger changes gradually, and you do not set yourself unrealistic targets. Criteria are changeable. Just because they are down on paper does not mean that they are there for ever. You can review them and change them as your circumstances change, or as the staff's knowledge increases, or for any other legitimate reason. As long as the change is approved in the same way as the original criteria – by discussion and agreement by all concerned. Your standards should be *dynamic*, and that means they should be constantly reviewed and improved where possible, or changed to cope with a changing environment. Do not be afraid of them – they are *yours* – and you know best how to keep them relevant and appropriate to your workplace.

At the end of this chapter you will be able to achieve the following:

● Choose which format to use for your standards

● Understand what is meant by structure, process and outcome criteria within the context of standard setting, and be able to differentiate between the three

● Construct criteria in simple sentences that are unambiguous, measurable, achievable and have been agreed by all involved

In short, you should be able to write a standard that is relevant to your work area.

CHAPTER 3

What to Do with Your Standard Once it is Written

It is only Chapter 3, and you have written a standard already. You have organised your group, brainstormed your ideas, clarified a standard statement, written down some specific structure, process and outcome criteria, and you have a written, agreed standard in front of you. So, what do you do with it now?

I regularly meet with nurses who have spent a great deal of their time and effort writing standards. They have been all fired up, meeting together and getting excited over what they can and cannot do, and drafting out a really good standard. When they have got it down on paper, they start on another one, and when they have got two, they start on a third. Pretty soon, they have a folder full of excellent standards, and slowly they begin to lose interest. After all, it is a lot of hard work isn't it? And just how many of these things do you need to have anyway? The folder sits on a shelf in the office, no one ever looks at it, but when the auditor comes round and asks if they have any standards they can say 'Yes, we've got all these'. Unfortunately, no one works to them, because no one looks at them; no one knows if they reflect the standard of care being carried out because no one has thought about monitoring them. In short, they are a waste of time. You have got fifteen standards in a folder – so what? If they are not being measured and reviewed, then you may as well have fifteen pieces of newspaper in your folder.

My advice is always to monitor your first standard before you start to write any more. It is very easy to get carried away with the standard writing – after all, it can be fun, it is an opportunity for you all to get together, it feels as though you are actually doing something, and that can feel very satisfying in itself. But, you must face up to monitoring straight away.

Try to see standard setting as being made up of three activities:

1. Writing the standard

2. Measuring the standard

3. Making any changes that need to be made.

These three activities together constitute standard setting and they cannot, and must not, be separated.

Think about it a little. What is the point of a written standard if you are not going to find out if you are meeting it or not? What is the point of finding out that you are not meeting the standard, if you are not going to do anything about it? And from the other way around – how can you take action to improve care if you do not know exactly what needs to be improved? Even more important in these times of being expected to audit your practice – how can you audit your practice if you have not identified what good practice is?

This seems very simple and straightforward, but you would be surprised at the number of people who do not connect standards with audit. How *do* you audit if you have not defined what it is that you expect to see? Standard setting is one very good way of getting to grips with audit in a very practical way so that it is relevant and useful to you in your own area, and so that it provides useful information to you and your managers.

If you want your standards to be taken seriously, then it is important that you think about some kind of approval mechanism for them within the organisation. You need them to be recognised as working documents that your Unit or Trust is committed to, not just 'something that the nurses do'. This is where you need to have your manager on board. Whether your managers belong to the same profession or not, they need to understand what you are doing, and they need to feel able to support you. You need to have your standards approved by the person or persons to whom you are managerially accountable and not just keep them at ward or department level or just take them through the professional structure. If you are really going to start making significant changes (and you might) you will need approval from the people who hold the purse strings and who have the organisational authority. They probably will not have the time to be involved in your standard-writing sessions, so participation in that sense may not be the answer. However, your best bet is to keep them informed – send them the drafts just as you do to other members of the team, and take notice of any comments that may be made. Let them see that you are being sensible, that you are not being idealistic, and that these standards can actually help them to get a better feel of how your patch works and what your values are. If you are sensitive, then the chances are that you will get approval of your standards without any difficulty at all. You may have to clarify one or two things, you may have to spend a little time explaining why you chose to have certain criteria, but at the end of the day it will be worth it to have management approval of your level of care. This is the first step towards bringing the whole of the team together, and really beginning to get that shared philosophy which you see written about in so many documents.

Now, back to the business of standard setting. You have written your standard, and you are going to monitor it. First of all, stop and take stock a minute. Is the standard that you have written down going to involve a period of implementation? For instance, say that you have written a standard about parents and children being well informed prior to admission for elective surgery. One of your structure criteria might be that there is a supply of relevant, up-to-date literature available for sending out to parents. However, the literature that you have at the moment is really awful – not geared to children at all, and written in a boring and patronising way. In fact, one of the main reasons for writing this standard was because you wanted to do something about the available literature, but no one ever seemed to get around to it. You might well want to review and make some changes to the literature before you monitor the standard. This, if you allocate it as a project to two or three specific members of staff, might take a couple of months, so you need an implementation period of a couple of months to get this in place before you start your monitoring process.

During this implementation period it is important that you continue to meet at the same regular intervals to keep an eye on the 'sub-group', to make sure that things are progressing and that everyone maintains their involvement. It is easy at this stage for people to begin to lose interest and those of you who are facilitating the process must keep things together and try to keep people motivated. Continuing feedback is really helpful for this, and if you are not actually a part of the ward team, do continue to visit the ward or department to check that everything is going to plan and to encourage the group.

If your standard is a reflection of good care that you are pretty sure is already happening, then you may not need an implementation period and you may want to monitor straight away, just to confirm your feelings, and give everyone some really positive feedback. (Then you will all be highly motivated to go on and write another standard because it is actually not as bad as you thought it was going to be!)

The standard-setting group will need to be prepared for monitoring their standard. Some people really do not like the idea of being monitored or watched or 'checked up on' – they feel quite threatened by it. If you have been sensitive right from the start and made sure that everyone understood that standard setting consists of three stages, one of which is monitoring, then you should not have too much of a problem. If you are acting as facilitator it will be up to you to try to make sure that your group feel as comfortable as possible about the monitoring phase. If they have all been involved in the setting of the standard and they understand what it is and how it works, then the chances are they will be quite looking forward to monitoring things and finding out how well they are doing. Rather than being threatened by the idea of monitoring, they are more likely to be concerned about the practicalities – just exactly how do they monitor this standard? Who will do it? How long will it take? What will they have to do?

Monitoring standards is not really as difficult as you might think. Basically there are two main methods that can be used:

- **Observing** – incorporating document checks, environmental checks, observing practice, observing interactions.

- **Asking questions** – incorporating asking nurses, patients, carers, other professionals, anyone relevant, either by questionnaire or by some kind of interview.

Observing

If you need to use the nursing documentation for your monitoring exercise (or any other kind of chart) you need to decide at what point in the patient's stay you need to obtain your information. Do you need to check it while the patient is still receiving care, that is, to look at it *concurrently* with care? Or can you 'pull' documentation after discharge and check through for specific information, that is, *retrospective* monitoring.

How feasible is it for you to use documentation at all for monitoring? If you do choose to use it, I guarantee that you will have to do some work on accuracy, timeliness and legibility! So, if you are planning to use documentation as a source of information, make sure that it is up to scratch before you start. Some off-the-shelf audit tools use documentation almost exclusively as their monitoring method. Think about your own nursing documentation – how accurate is it? How 'good' is it as a source of information? Can you guarantee that you will be able to find the same sort of information in every care plan – and not just the demographic stuff from the front page? An audit is only as good as the information it collects: if your documentation is unreliable, then your results will be unreliable too.

Still on 'observing' – what about observing practice? Observing one's colleagues is always tricky. First of all, do you observe people covertly, so they do not realise that you are watching them? This way you will get a true picture of what is going on, but you will probably lose some friends and be extremely unpopular. Or do you observe overtly, so that everyone knows that you will be observing them and is ready for it? Do you go for participant observation – that is, do you observe your colleagues' activities whilst you are working alongside them? Or do you go for non-participant observation where you observe without joining in the work? There are advantages and disadvantages with all of these. As mentioned previously – covert observation needs ethical consideration. Is it right to monitor your colleagues' work without telling them? How would you feel if it happened to you? I personally have never carried out any truly covert observation – simply because I feel a bit uncomfortable about it.

But what about overt observation? Surely if everyone knows that they are being observed, then they are going to alter their behaviour so that you see what they want you to see? Well, yes, this does happen – people often do perform better when they are being watched, or they are more careful than usual, or whatever. However, there are ways around this problem. Most people get used to being observed very quickly – within a couple of days they are back to normal behaviour whether being watched or not. The simplest solution is to observe quite openly for say, five days, and then discard the observations from the first two days. It is reasonable to expect that by the third day normal behaviour will be resumed! Obviously you will have to work out the timescales to suit yourself and your own situations, but this is one way around that difficulty.

To participate or not to participate? Being a participant observer is great, you get to be a part of the team, help with the work, and make your observations at the same time. You are not in the way, you are contributing as a worker and it can be very satisfying for everyone. Unfortunately it is quite hard to do this. My own problem with being a participant observer is that I tend to get so involved with the work in hand (not having as many opportunities for clinical work as I would like), that I forget to observe and miss something vital. You might also find that, as with overt observation, the mere fact that you are working alongside the person you are observing makes them modify their behaviour – your presence may affect the results.

Being a non-participant observer is frankly very tedious. Even if you spend time preparing for it and everyone forgets that you are there observing, you still feel like a spare part. And what do you do if a patient asks you to do something for them – while you are just standing there 'doing nothing'? Do you forget the observations and do it? Do you forget the observations while you find someone else to do it? Do you try to keep observing while you do whatever it is?

Non-participant observation when done for any length of time can be very boring – it is not uncommon to find yourself day-dreaming or writing the shopping list or wondering why Sister So and So does not clean her shoes more often. This is called observer drift and it happens to everybody at some point or another. You will have to weigh up all these pros and cons with your own situation and decide, preferably with your group, which is the best way to obtain the information that you want and which is the method that most people feel most comfortable with.

Asking questions

Questionnaires

Whenever we need to obtain information from individuals, the ubiquitous questionnaire always emerges. For some reason it appears to be everyone's first choice – probably because at first sight it seems so convenient. Think really hard before you opt for a written questionnaire. First of all, they are actually quite difficult to construct so that you get the information that you want. Secondly, there are problems of timing – when do you ask people to fill them in?

If you are expecting patients to respond to questionnaires, do you give them out while they are in hospital or do you wait until they have gone home? Giving them out in hospital saves time and postage and so on, but it may mean that the patients do not feel able to say what they really think because they are still being looked after by you. If you wait until after discharge, they may not bother to reply at all, being only too glad to be at home and feeling better. Or their views may be tempered by the distance of being at home and they 'forget' all the criticisms that they had while they were with you.

If you send questionnaires out by post and expect a return by post, expect a very small return – perhaps as small as 20 per cent. Expect to have to remind people at least once. And expect to have to be very organised indeed. Should you use a stamped addressed envelope or a reply-paid envelope? Someone once told me, and unfortunately I cannot remember who, always to use a stamp – people will ignore a reply-paid official envelope, but they are less likely to waste a stamp! I am not sure if this is strictly true, but anything that increases your return rate is worth a try!

There are other problems that arise when you choose the written reply to a questionnaire as your method. You immediately exclude anyone who cannot read or write. You exclude anyone who cannot read or write English, unless your documents are multilingual. You are probably excluding children.

If you want to ascertain the level of nurses' knowledge about something, rather than obtain an opinion from a patient, then you need to be very careful, not only about how you frame the questions, but also the whole approach. You do not want people to feel as though they are resitting their Final Examinations all over again. Be sensitive.

If you feel that the questionnaire is the only way for you, then please get some expert help with it. Getting the questions right, and getting the information that you need, in a format that is usable, often requires expert assistance.

There are a number of different ways of conducting an interview – they can be structured and very formal, where each person is asked exactly the same question with no prompting or assistance from the interviewer. Or they can run through varying degrees of formality, right down to the friendly chat.

The problems are similar to those with questionnaires – do you interview patients while they are in hospital or receiving care – risking that they may be less than honest in case it affects their care later, or because they are so grateful for your ministrations that the most awful care would be deemed wonderful? Do you wait until they go home and then struggle with the logistical difficulties of interviewing people in their own homes – travelling expenses, time, making convenient appointments, and so on? Could you interview over the telephone – excluding people automatically who do not have a phone, who do not speak English, who are deaf, who are dysphasic? In addition to these, you would also be missing out on any non-verbal clues.

Could you do a sort of 'exit' interview – speaking to people just as they are about to leave or be discharged from your care? All of these are possibilities and may be suitable depending on your situation.

The actual interviewing process can be fraught with difficulty. Again, it is helpful if you have some expertise in this particular method, or if you have access to someone who can give you some help. In a semi-structured interview, which is quite a good format to use, you need to be able to paraphrase your questions if they are not understood, you need to be able to pick up on non-verbal clues and encourage people to say a little more if you think it necessary. You do need to be able to relate easily to the people you are interviewing – stilted conversations are embarrassing and often may not give you the information you really want. You may have to plan your interviews so that you can spend a little time just chatting and putting your interviewees at their ease. Do not forget to build in time for this kind of thing.

Consider how you are going to record the interview data that you collect. Will you be able to make notes as you interview? Might it be a bit off-putting for the interviewees to have you scribbling away in front of them? Saying, 'Hang on a minute, I didn't quite get that bit'. Writing down responses in an interview is not the best way. You *can* do it – if you can do shorthand then it is feasible to do things this way, but even then you have to translate it all back and be sure that you have translated things accurately.

The obvious answer is to use a tape recorder for interviewing. There are some problems however, as some people may not like the idea of being recorded. How can you reassure them that the tapes will be confidential and for your ears only? As mentioned before, some people will be embarrassed by being recorded – you will have to spend a little time just chatting to get them relaxed and responding freely. If you can get people to agree to being recorded then it is a very good way of accurately recording your interviews and of being sure that you are not going to miss anything. Obvious points to remember are always to make sure that your batteries are good or that you have a suitable mains electricity connector, and to take more tapes than you are planning on using. If people need time to pause and think before replying, you cannot keep turning the tape on and off! Once it is set and running, then it stays running until the interview is finished.

This is by no means an exhaustive look at monitoring methods, but I think it is probably enough to get you started and to get you thinking. Do not be afraid to try out these methods – there is nothing mysterious about them. There are books much more in depth than this that you can turn to when you are ready to refine your activity a little. With practice you will find the best way of doing things.

At the end of this chapter you will be able to:

● State the three stages of standard setting – writing the standard, monitoring the standard and taking action, and that these three stages must not be separated

● Explain the importance of having an approval mechanism for your standards which includes management approval

● Recognise when standards may need an implementation period

● Identify the most commonly used methods of monitoring and some of their advantages and disadvantages.

CHAPTER 4

Monitoring your Standard (1)

(The following chapters on monitoring use a modified and simplified version of the audit method currently promoted by the Royal College of Nursing Dynamic Quality Improvement Programme.)

At this point you should have a standard in front of you ready to be monitored. You will have an idea of the main monitoring methods that you might use, and some of the problems that may arise. But in practical terms, what do you do next? First, give some thought to deciding which part of the standard you need to monitor.

There are three columns of criteria in front of you – structure, process and outcome. Which of these should you be interested in measuring? There is a school of thought that suggests we should concentrate our measurement efforts on outcomes only – if we monitor the outcomes and we seem to be achieving them, then the theory is that everything must be alright. Also in favour of outcomes only is the fact that you probably have just three or four outcomes in your standard so it should not take too long to complete the monitoring procedure. Unfortunately, it is not quite as simple as this.

What are the problems associated with monitoring just the outcome column? First of all, what will that monitoring tell us? It *should* tell us whether the outcomes have been met or not. And if we have met them we can relax. Or can we? How do we know that we met the outcomes as a result of the other elements of the standard? How will we know if the rest of the standard had anything to do with it at all? We may have reached those outcomes *in spite* of what we did, not *because* of what we did. We may have achieved them quite by chance. Monitoring outcomes alone will not tell us how we got to that point.

What if we did not meet the outcomes? How will we know where we went wrong? All we will know is that the outcomes have not been met. Why were they not met? What do we have to work on to put things right? Unfortunately, just monitoring the outcomes does not give us any information about where we might need to do some extra work.

One of the main reasons for going to all the trouble of writing standards in this particular way is so that when we monitor we can say: 'We think that these things happen – these outcomes are reached – because we have these things (structures), and because we do these things (processes); and if we don't have these structures, or if we cannot undertake these particular processes, then this will probably have a bearing on our outcomes'. If we are only monitoring outcomes, then we cannot track back through our standard like this and make this point to our managers. We cannot relate our structures and processes to the outcomes if we have not monitored them at the same time and looked for possible connections. An outcome may be meaningless unless we can relate it to a preceding process. If we *can* relate it to a preceding process then we can repeat that process and hope to ensure the same outcome. Conversely, we can stop doing the things that do not seem to produce a positive outcome.

Therefore, unless we monitor both process *and* outcome and their links, we are not making best use of all this work.

So far we have not mentioned anything about structures – do they need to be monitored as well? The answer
is 'Yes, they do', particularly for new standards where
you may have made your structure requirements explicit
for the first time. But if you think about it, most of the
things in your structures are fairly static once they are in
place – equipment, facilities, knowledge base, and so on.
So, perhaps structures do not have to be monitored quite
so often as the other two sets of criteria. But remember,
this is just my opinion – you must decide for yourself
based on the conditions that you work in.

For the first monitoring of your standard, I would suggest that you monitor everything – every structure, process and outcome. After that, it will be self-evident where
you need to take action and where you need to remonitor.
But at the first attempt – MONITOR ALL YOUR CRITE-
RIA. It will give you a very clear picture of what is going on with that particular standard and it will give you
some very clear pointers as to the action you need to
take.

So, back to that standard which you have in front of
you. You now know the importance of monitoring all
criteria, but what exactly do you need to do? Remember
in Chapter 3 we discussed various methods of monitoring, such as checking documentation, observing practice,
asking nurses, and so on? Now you need to decide which
of these methods you will use to monitor your standard.

Consider the first criterion in your structure column –
how might you monitor it? Think of the example of
'parents going to the anaesthetic room'. This standard is
shown in full in Figure 4.1. The first structure criterion
states:

*The pre-theatre room is geared to receiving children and there
are toys and books available.*

How can we find out if this is actually the case? We

41

Figure 4.1
Standard Setting Text

STANDARD STATEMENT: ALL PARENTS OR GUARDIANS HAVE THE OPPORTUNITY TO ACCOMPANY THEIR CHILD INTO THE PRE-OPERATIVE WARD OR ANAESTHETIC ROOM		
STRUCTURE	PROCESS	OUTCOME
S1 The Pre-Operative ward is geared to receiving parents and children. There are toys and books available.	P1 A trained nurse explains to each parent/guardian that they may accompany their child to the pre-operative ward/anaesthetic room if they wish to do so.	01 Every child and parent is received into a relaxed, calm environment.
S2 All anaesthetic staff are fully aware of the child's needs and there are 'safe' staffing levels to cater for this.	P2 Parents or guardians are given a brief explanation of their role in the pre-operative ward/ anaesthetic room.	02 Every parent/guardian who wishes to accompany their child to the pre-operative ward/anaesthetic room, has the opportunity to do so.
S3 The paediatric recovery area is separate from the pre-operative ward.	P3 Parents are accepted into the anaesthetic room with the co-operation of the anaesthetist.	
S4 Overshoes, hats and gowning facilities are available for parents if required.	P4 Safety aspects of theatre area are briefly explained to parents/ guardians.	

could go and look, to see if the room is geared to children and if there are actually toys and books there for the children to use. Therefore, this criterion can be monitored by direct observation. We therefore visit the theatre area and check out the pre-theatre facilities against our criterion.

Now consider the first process criterion in the same standard.

The nurse explains to the parent that he or she may attend the pre-theatre room or anaesthetic room if he or she wishes to do so.

How can we monitor this criterion? There are two different approaches that we could take here. First, we could observe the nurse as she gives information to the patient, noting if she actually imparts this particular piece of information. Secondly, we might wait until the child is ready to be discharged and then talk to the parents about their experience. We can ask the parents then if they were told they could go to the pre-operative room if they had wanted to. So we have a choice of direct observation or interview/questionnaire. In fact we have three possibilities: the third possibility is that we could use both methods together – we could observe to see if the nurse gives the information and we can cross-check this by subsequently asking the parents if they were given this information. Cross-checking in this way can be quite helpful – for instance, we might observe that the nurse gives the correct information to the parents, but when we ask the parents they may state they were not told. This might be a simple case of forgetfulness, or it might mean that they do not remember the information because it was given at an inappropriate time – when the parents were particularly anxious, for instance, or when they were distracted by their frightened child, or perhaps the nurses' manner was such that they did not really register the information. You will see from Figure 4.2 how two questions and methods have been used to check out this criterion. In fact this 'double-check' method has been used for a number of the criteria in this standard.

So, what about the second structure criterion?:

Nurses in the pre-theatre room are aware of the child's possible needs prior to surgery and there are 'safe' staffing levels to cater for this.

How are we going to know if the theatre staff are aware of the needs of children? We shall have to ask them. It is therefore necessary to decide the essential things that

Figure 4.2
Standard Setting Text

AUDITOR:

DATE OF AUDIT:

METHOD	CODE	AUDIT CRITERIA
Check Environment	S1a	Is the pre-op ward geared to receiving children?
	S1b	Are there toys and books available in the pre-op ward?
	S2b	In your opinion, are there sufficient staff on duty for the environment to be considered 'safe'?
	S3	Is the paediatric recovery area separate from the pre-op ward?
	S4	Are overshoes, hats and gowns available for parents?
Ask nurses	S2a	Can each nurse caring for children in the anaesthetic room/ pre-theatre ward give a brief description of the likely needs of children prior to surgery?
Ask parents	P1	Has each parent been told that they may accompany their child to pre-theatre/anaesthetic room?
	P2a	Has each parent been told what is expected of them in the pre-theatre/anaesthetic room?
	P2b	Can each parent say what those expectations are?
	P4a	Has each parent been told about the safety aspects of pre-theatre/anaesthetic room?
	P4b	Can each parent briefly describe the safety aspects?
	O3	Was each parent who expressed a wish to accompany their child to pre-theatre/anaesthetic room allowed to do so?
	01 & 02	Give each parent the opportunity to discuss whether visiting the pre-theatre/anaesthetic room made them feel less anxious or helped them in any way. Make a note of main comments.

theatre staff need to be aware of regarding children prior to theatre, and then ask them to tell us about them.

But what about 'safe' staffing levels? What does this mean? Isn't 'Safe' one of those taboo words that are not supposed to appear in standards? This criterion is from a standard that is used by a group of nurses on a busy paediatric unit. They themselves chose to use the term – but they had to decide what it meant first. They did not want to put a number in that criterion because it would alter from day to day – some days two nurses might be enough, on other days they might need six, so to use a particular number would limit them. They concluded that the answer was to take account of the number of children in the theatre area, their condition and proposed surgery, and then to compare this with the number of staff on duty. It was agreed the paediatric nurse specialist would do this, before making a judgement about whether she considered these to be 'safe' staffing levels or not. The specialist nurse's professional judgement was agreed as the best way of judging a changing situation. So, the method of measurement for this criterion is direct observation and clinical judgement.

It is straightforward isn't it? Just use the same approach with each of the criteria in the standard. That is, identify a monitoring method (or more than one if necessary) for each of the criteria in the structure, process and outcome columns.

What you will find is that it may not always be immediately obvious which method of measuring is most appropriate. This usually means that your criteria have not been written specifically enough and not in really measurable terms. If this is the case, then your questions will be really difficult to construct, finding a way of obtaining a yes/no answer will be difficult and the whole business will feel drawn out and complicated. My experience has been that the first attempt at measurement often tells you more about your standard-writing technique than it does about the quality of your care! In fact, you can often consider your first measurement as being like a pilot study – it will help to point out any mistakes or problems with your technique before you go on to accept the standard as a working document. You can then refine the standard criteria before you measure again – making sure that they are more relevant, specific and measurable this time. There are not really any short cuts to this in the early stages. You almost need to make these mistakes in order to understand the best way of constructing the criteria and how you need to think about them in the future. Do not be too concerned about this at this stage, as mentioned earlier on in this book, it does get easier with practice – it is a literacy skill that can be learned.

Well constructed, clear and specific criteria are the key to good standard setting, you just have to keep trying them out until they work.

Figure 4.2 gives an example of monitoring questions for the paediatric standard. Note how each question is really just the criterion turned around. Also note how each set of criteria are grouped together under their monitoring method so that you can deal with them all at the same time. You can organise yourself so that you are not flitting from an observation to a question to a documentation check.

In order to keep your paperwork to a minimum (remembering that your standard should really be as short as you can reasonably make it), you can place your audit questions on the reverse side of your standard. In this way the two are always together, and you have the standard handy to refer to if necessary when you are auditing.

In these last two chapters, basic monitoring methods have been briefly discussed. Although this has been at an elementary level, it should be sufficient to get you started and give you some idea of how you can begin to audit in a sensible and practical way. As you become more familiar with these simple monitoring techniques, you will find yourself wanting to find out more about the methods you are using, and how to apply them perhaps a little more rigorously. The important thing at this stage is to get a feel for these simple techniques and not try to do too much too quickly. A simple snapshot view is all you require and this kind of exercise will provide you with that. You will become more sophisticated about monitoring once you have mastered basic techniques and you begin to feel confident about applying these methods in this simple way. Once you have tried them out you will see how such relatively simple approaches can provide you with useful data upon which you can act.

If you are reading this book as a facilitator, or potential facilitator, there are some points to remember. It is very disheartening for a group to find, as they often do, that their criteria are unmeasurable and they have to rewrite much of their standard. Your job is to point this out as tactfully as possible, and, at first, to offer alternative forms of words. You may well think that a lot of time may have been saved if you had given more direction with criteria construction in the first place, but this process of learning by mistakes is extremely fruitful. There is a great deal of satisfaction in hearing the group you are working with begin to question how measurable their criteria are as they write them.

Facilitation is complex and there is a fine line between allowing learning through mistakes and letting the group muddle on without help. The learning experience should be positive whenever possible. This is the responsibility of every facilitator and the skill of a good one.

At the end of this chapter you will be able to:

● Discuss why it is important to measure all your criteria – structure, process and outcome – when you monitor for the first time

● Identify which monitoring method best suits each criterion

● Explain how monitoring can be made easier by refining any vague criteria

● Convert each criterion into a simple question requiring a yes/no answer

● Group these questions together according to the monitoring method being used

● Devise a simple format for keeping your questions together with the written standard.

CHAPTER 5

Monitoring Your Standard (2)

Having written a standard, and developed a simple monitoring tool (the what, how and who of auditing), the next stage is to consider 'how many' or, how big does our sample for auditing need to be? Having considered what or who needs to be monitored and having considered that our monitoring may involve asking nurses or patients questions, how many nurses or patients should we ask? Alternatively, if choosing to monitor by observing particular interactions or interventions, how many episodes do we need to watch? Therefore what should the sample size be?

How big does a sample need to be? Are large numbers needed to give the study credibility? One hundred patients? Two hundred? Observe one hundred interventions? Just how long will such an audit take and how much time? How will interest be maintained? Is it really necessary to have such large numbers?

It is important to remember that we are interested in *audit* – in finding out what is happening to a group of patients and how they feel about it. We are not undertaking a piece of research, we are not trying to prove a hypothesis, or demonstrate a causal relationship. We *are* trying to find out what is happening on one ward, to one particular group of patients, being cared for by one particular group of nurses. This audit is for our own local purposes and for our own local clients. This means that our sample size does not need to be huge. One of the main reasons why sample sizes need to be large in some research studies is that the researchers often want to generalise their results – they want to be able to say that what happened to the subjects in their study is likely to happen to other subjects if the study is repeated. This claim can really only be made if the sample size is large and representative of the relevant population and the findings relate to a significant proportion of that population. The larger the sample is, the easier it is to make the calculations and to assess the significance. This is something of a simplistic explanation, but sample size and generalisability are connected. For audit purposes, as said before, we do not want to generalise our findings – we are only interested in these few patients on one ward. It makes sense therefore, not to worry too much about small sample sizes. The important point is that the sample size is adequate (in your opinion) to reflect the common characteristics of your client group. You will, however, need to pay some attention to choosing the content of your sample.

Think back to the beginning of the book when we were first thinking about writing a standard. We had to decide who the standard was applicable to – who was the 'client group'. For instance, in our anaesthetic room standard, it was all children for elective surgery. 'All children for elective surgery' is the client group. This means that the sample for our audit has to come from that particular client group – the sample will consist of children who are going to theatre and their parents. There is no point in us asking the particular questions in our audit tool of parents whose children are not going to go to theatre, it would be irrelevant. Likewise, in our teaching standard for patients with diabetes, the sample group would need to be new patients with diabetes who were capable of learning how to check their own blood sugar.

So, the first identifier of our sample is the specific client group that the standard is aimed at. Depending on the nature of your standard this may be a huge number of clients, or a very small number. If it is a small number, this can actually make things easier for you. Take our diabetic teaching standard – on a general medical ward in a smallish general hospital, you may not get many new diabetic patients coming for teaching. It may be as few as one or two in a month. In this case, how do you organise your audit so that you capture a reasonable number of patients? What if you decide to audit all new diabetic patients over a one-month period and there are none in the month that you have chosen to audit? In this case you need to think about the number of clients that is likely to be available and the number of clients that you think give a reasonable idea of how the standard was working. Look back through your records. Last year your ward provided care for thirty new diabetic patients, admitted for stabilisation and education. So the total you can expect is thirty, and that would take about a year to audit. Too long. Audit needs to be about quick turn-round of information. You could decide to monitor all new diabetics who come in for stabilisation and education until you have audited fifteen. That's fifty per cent of your expected population and it should not take quite so long to work through them.

Consider the parents and anaesthetic room standard. The client group here is all children for elective surgery – that is going to be a much higher number, probably at least fifteen per week. This would be an awful lot of work in a very short space of time. So, think about choosing your sample in a different way from saying 'all parents whose children are having elective surgery'. You could for example, monitor every fifth set of parents whose child was having elective surgery until you had monitored twenty sets of parents. In this way you would probably be looking at two or three per week. This is much more manageable, and it would spread the work over a couple of months. Your sample size will depend on how big your client group is, and on how long you are prepared to wait to obtain some results. With a very small client group you will have to wait a longer time in order to get a reasonable number. Auditing one client out of an annual population of thirty is not really going to be very helpful. Use your common sense – the smaller the client group the longer the collection of data will take, the larger the client group the faster the data collection. Do not however, be tempted not to write standards for, or audit, aspects of care that occur very infrequently or for a very small number of patients. One person's opinion, even if it is the only opinion you are likely to have, is valid. I would suggest however, that you do not audit these very small client groups for the first time around – you will feel as if you are doing an awful lot of work for a very small result, and that can be quite demotivating!

Apart from sample size, there may be other considerations. How do you choose who to include and who to leave out of your audit? You may have to exclude some patients from your audit – especially if your potential sample population is very large and you simply can not cope with auditing everyone. Also, your audit tool may automatically exclude some clients. For example, if sending a questionnaire to patients following discharge to their home address, this will automatically exclude people who cannot read, particularly people who cannot read English. If your audit tool relies upon interviewing patients then any patient who is unconscious, or who may be away from the ward on the day of the audit will also be excluded.

You may want to make deliberate exclusions. For example, if you are trying to find out how well elderly people respond to education concerning their diabetes you may want to exclude everyone below a certain age, say sixty-five years old. If you wanted to compare the results for this group with a younger age group, you would undertake exactly the same audit, but this time you would exclude all those over sixty-five. Again, think about it logically, apply a bit of common sense and you will not make many mistakes.

A good facilitator will encourage groups to think more carefully about sample sizes and exclusions as they become more experienced. In the early stages it can be confusing to have to think about all this as well as getting the criteria right and developing a sensible monitoring tool. Sometimes it is easier at the beginning to be fairly arbitrary about samples and so on, until confidence is built up. There will be a point in the proceedings when sample size will occur to someone as perhaps needing more than a consideration of numbers, and then off you go into a whole new stage of development, and a deeper knowledge of techniques and methods will be required, learned about and tried out in practice. Learning in stages like this, and at the group's own pace – not the facilitator's – will mean that the lessons are learned well and are understood as they are used. My own experience of working with groups has shown that this does happen, that learning does take place often without people realising it. The satisfaction is the facilitator's when someone says 'So that's what they mean when they talk about choosing a sample . . .', or 'Hang on a minute, wouldn't it be better if we left out all those patients with such and such, and just concentrated on these?'

'What', 'how' and 'how many' are behind us. So is 'who', in terms of who gets monitored. Now we need to think about who *does* the monitoring. At the very beginning of this book we discussed the importance of nurses being involved in setting standards. We talked about how important it is that nurses have a sense of ownership of their standards and that participating in writing and agreeing them can result in that ownership. The same principle applies to auditing standards. In order to achieve any change, the people who are going to have to bring about that change need to understand why it is needed. They need to have worked out for themselves where the problems are, and what the solutions might be. Participating in audit is fundamental to obtaining ownership of audit results and increasing the likelihood of action being taken. In the past, wherever I have worked with groups of nurses on standard setting and improving their practice, it is the same nurses who have audited their own standards. It makes sense for those involved to work their way through the whole cycle of events.

There are two main approaches to undertaking audit: *internally*, as I have just explained, where those involved audit themselves; and *externally* – where someone quite independent undertakes the audit part of the cycle and feeds back to those being audited. Both approaches have their place and both can be of equal value.

If you decide to use internal auditing methods – and I strongly advise you to do this when you first start, for all the reasons given earlier – then you need to be aware of certain pitfalls. So, what are the disadvantages of monitoring your own practice? The main problem is bias. It stands to reason that there is always the possibility that you may not be as objective as you should be when your own standards, your own colleagues, or your own friends are under your scrutiny. Will you turn a blind eye if you see something you do not like? Will you ignore someone's behaviour on one occasion because you know it is out of character, and at any other time it would not have happened? Will you choose to undertake your audit on a day when it is very quiet and everything can be done absolutely perfectly? Or will you choose a day when all hell is let loose and you know the audit will look dreadful? (Motives for undertaking audit can vary widely, and be open to all kinds of manipulation if you want it to be!). Bias is the one challenge that is always raised whenever I have talked about nurses monitoring their own standards. I maintain the argument that it is necessary for nurses to go through and understand every part of the standard-setting/audit process if they are to take it, and the results of it, seriously. I also have to add, that in six years of working with nurses on setting and auditing standards I have never known any of them to 'cheat' on their monitoring – never. For one thing, a good facilitator gets to know his/her groups very well, and knows when they are ready to really examine what they are doing – warts and all. Most groups will nominate someone from within their number to undertake the monitoring process for them. Often someone will volunteer. If they are particularly nervous about the techniques, or about the time it might take, then they may ask the facilitator to undertake the monitoring for them. Some groups expect the facilitator to do the monitoring. I personally try to discourage this as it does not encourage groups to get involved. But, if there are problems with getting to grips with the techniques, or if there are serious time constraints or workload constraints, then I have willingly helped groups to do their monitoring. Normally, by this time, the facilitator is seen as part of the group anyway, and no one feels threatened or bothered by it. It should be emphasised though, that the best way forward is for a member of the working group from the ward to undertake the audit. It does not need to be the Ward Sister (this may, in fact, be intimidating for some people). It can be anyone who is willing, and who understands what needs to be done. The facilitator's role here is to support and guide, not take over and do.

Occasionally, there is a strong feeling that the risk of bias is unacceptable and that some form of external monitoring should take place, objectivity usually being given as the prime reason. This is perfectly acceptable, but again, consideration needs to be given to who does this monitoring. If it is a senior person, say the nurse manager or senior clinical nurse for the unit, then the nurses being monitored may feel intimidated or even worried about negative bias. At the end of the day, a lot of this kind of problem comes down to personalities, and to trust. If the relationships between people are not good, then bringing them together for audit purposes can feel punitive or inspectorial – exactly the opposite of what we really want.

For me, the biggest difficulty with using external auditors in the early stages lies in the lack of mutual understanding. Often if standards are written about particular and very specific problems, the monitoring will require an understanding of the nuances and undercurrents of the ward in order to make the best interpretation. A 'stranger', with the best will in the world, will not be able to do this. They may be scrupulously fair, but they may miss something that an internal auditor would not, and that something may be fundamental to the outcome of the audit.

An external auditor, in order to do the job as well as possible, is going to need very careful preparation. He or she will need a clear understanding of the purpose of the standard and of the audit. The audit questions will need to be absolutely clear and the criteria they refer to unambiguous. The instructions about who to ask questions, or where to look for certain things have to be absolutely clear. There is no room at all for possible interpretations with an external auditor, it all must be totally straightforward and black and white. External auditing is really for when you feel that you have seriously got your act together.

In the early stages, when developing an understanding of the process and its benefits is arguably more important than the quality of the result, then an internal auditor wins for me, every time.

Having said that, when everyone is used to the idea and knows what is happening, and feels OK about it all, then a sensitive external auditor may be the right way to proceed. It will reduce bias, it will give other people more confidence in your results, and it will mean that you can obtain more feedback, not just on the audit but on other related issues that the external auditor, with fresh eyes, may have picked up.

If I can refer to my own experience again – the groups I have worked with have been very keen to undertake their own auditing early on. They enter into it with enthusiasm the first few times, but they soon realise that it is a tedious, time-consuming task that takes them away from other things. Soon they start asking for different ways of undertaking the audit – such as asking someone else to do it. I have known groups nominate someone on a rotating basis from within their number, I have known them to rely on their senior nurse or nurse specialist to do it. I have known groups ask colleagues from similar wards to undertake the audit for them and to loan the helping ward a member of staff while it is being done. Using colleagues from other wards is a good way of progressing your audit process – it shows you have confidence in your own practice and are not afraid of scrutiny. It also means that there is some automatic sharing of practice and that you are beginning to take the first tentative steps toward peer review. An extremely exciting step to arise out of simple expediency! I am constantly heartened at how nurses move smoothly from one level of development to another, taking new and difficult concepts in their stride once they are on this pathway. (I am sorry if that sounds a bit trite, but it really does happen, and it really does make me feel as if I have been a part of something significant!)

In undertaking a nursing or clinical audit in the workplace, these five chapters provide you with the necessary guidance and explanations to make a start. The stages, as worked through previously, are as follows:

1. Deciding exactly what it is that you want to monitor or improve (identify topic)
2. Deciding what it is about this that you want to make different, and stating quite clearly how you want it to be (write a standard statement)
3. Describing all the details that are required in order for the standard statement to be realised (construct structure, process and outcome criteria)
4. Turning each of the criteria into a simple question that can be answered 'yes' or 'no', taking into consideration the method you would need to employ to answer each question (construct a simple audit tool)
5. Choosing the subjects you need to monitor – they may be people, interventions, environmental conditions – and how many of each one will give you a meaningful result (choosing the sample)
6. Trying out the monitoring tool by using it on a small scale – this will help identify any problems with the audit tool and the original standard (pilot study)
7. Deciding when to monitor seriously, who is going to do the monitoring and how long it is likely to take. Planning for this and making sure that everyone is prepared for it.

CHAPTER 6

Getting Results (1)

In the last two chapters we have considered monitoring methods and sampling. You should be able to decide which methods are best to use in which circumstances and how extensive your audit needs to be. There should be two or three simple papers in front of you – your standard and your monitoring tool with the questions on it.

It is now time to start thinking practically: how are you going to work through these questions so that you obtain sensible information, and so that the information you do get can be easily assimilated and acted upon? In the previous chapters we have discussed briefly some of the problems associated with monitoring techniques. However, it is worth revisiting some of this material again. Planning data collection is quite a long way from actually doing it and having an idea of what to expect can be useful.

At this point it will be helpful to return, briefly, to methods. Previously we considered asking questions – either by interview or questionnaire; we considered observation – overt and covert, participative and non-participative; and we considered some sort of environmental checking – documentation checking (chart audit) or looking at the environment of care. Collecting data using each of these methods need not be problematic if you are well prepared.

I would suggest you start with the 'asking questions'

methods. Earlier on in this book I mentioned making sure you grouped your audit questions together by method. For example, all questions for nurses are grouped together so that they can be asked at the same time; all questions for patients or relatives are grouped together; all observations requiring the auditor to look around the clinical environment are grouped together and so on. This simply keeps things neatly organised and will help you carry out your audit more efficiently.

Remember the points made in Chapter 3 about problems associated with different methods – I suggest that you go back to that chapter and re-read it now. With these potential difficulties fresh in your mind, it will help you to think very practically about the mechanics of data collection.

Whatever methods of data collection you plan to use, you will need to record your findings somewhere. If you are asking nurses or patients to fill in questionnaires then of course, the initial recording is done by the subject as they write in their answers. But, once everyone has responded, you will have ten or twenty, or even more, separate questionnaires in front of you – what are you going to do with them all? How are you going to start to make sense of the data?

If you have interviewed people and recorded those interviews and transcribed them, then you really do have a daunting prospect in front of you. A one-hour interview may turn out to be twenty or more closely typed sheets of paper. You may have ten or more transcribed interviews to deal with. Where are you going to start? Do not feel overwhelmed by the amount of information that you have in front of you. You will need to find a way of analysing and summarising it.

For the returned questionnaires it can be quite simple. Look at Figure 6.1, the summary sheet for the paediatric 'parent in the pre-operative room' standard. Draw up a grid on a large piece of paper. Put the question numbers

Figure 6.1
Standard Setting Text

ALL PARENTS ARE GIVEN THE OPPORTUNITY TO ACCOMPANY THEIR
CHILD TO THE PRE-THEATRE/ANAESTHETIC ROOM

SAMPLE:

AUDITOR:

DATE OF AUDIT:

CODE														TOTALS		COMMENTS
	1	2	3	4	5	6	7	8	9	10	11	12	13	YES	NO	
S1a																
S1b																
S2b																
S3																
S4																
S2a																
P1a																
P2a																
P2b																
P4a																
P4b																
03																
01 & 02																

or codes down the left-hand side and the respondent's
code or number across the top. For example, respondent
1, 2, 3, and so on. Fill in 'Y' for yes or 'N' for no in each
square depending on how they answered the question;
alternatively, use a tick or a cross. When you have done
this for every question, total up your 'Y's and 'N's (or
your ticks and crosses) and you have your first set of
results. If you process one questionnaire at a time, transferring all the answers on to your summary sheet, you
will not be leafing through all the papers for each separate question. At the end of the exercise you will have
all the information neatly contained on one piece of paper
plainly in front of you. In doing this you will see why it
is so important to frame your questions so that you can
obtain Yes or No answers. Anything other than Yes or
No and your simple grid summary sheet is not very useful.

I strongly recommend this Yes/No approach as the simplest to use, and Figure 6.1 gives an example of how it might look.

Sometimes you will find that even when you specifically ask for Yes or No answers, some respondents will still supply a short narrative if they feel particularly strongly about something. What you have to do here is note the extra information and which question it relates to. Do not ignore it. This kind of unsolicited material can be really helpful when you are interpreting your results and it can be very useful to include the odd quotation in your written report, as it adds some life to the statistics. For example, you may have asked patients a question about how the nurses gave information about their treatment. You may have asked:

'Were you satisfied with the explanations of your treatment given by the nursing staff?'

Ten people may have responded 'Yes' and two people responded 'No'. Of the ten who said 'Yes', one may have added 'I was lucky enough to be able to understand the language used, but someone else may not have'. This is a positive response formally, but it has a negative rider with it. The two people who gave negative responses may not have added anything to their simple 'No' response. Could there be a possibility that they were not satisfied because they could not understand what was being asked of them? You may want to follow this up with a quick telephone call or a subsequent chat if the patient is still with you. The rider from the one person may well have given you a lead to the reasons for the negative answers. Imagine if everyone who responded had simply put 'Yes' or 'No'. You would know that two people were not satisfied, but unless you had included a supplementary question, you would not have the faintest idea why.

It seems a little contradictory, doesn't it? On the one

hand you want 'Yes' or 'No' answers to keep things simple for you, but on the other hand some supplementary information can make a big difference to your interpretation of the results. There will always be some problems with questionnaires, however hard you try. Do try to obtain the help of an expert, or someone with some previous experience.

Returning to the main business of explaining how to use a summary sheet for collating the information you have collected – if you have interviewed people and have a number of transcribed interviews, this is more complicated to deal with, although it follows the same principles as the summary sheet. You obviously cannot make a simple grid, because respondents are not answering 'Yes' or 'No' to your questions. They are giving you a whole series of sentences back and you cannot fit that into a little square!

Dealing with transcripts takes much more time. You have to read through each one carefully, and begin to see where respondents are saying similar things in response to questions. You can highlight these similar responses with a coloured highlighter, the same colour for the similar response in each transcript. As you start to do this, you will begin to see that a lot of the responses begin to fit under broader headings, so you can start to make a list of the broader headings with the specific comment noted below it. This drawing out of similar information and grouping it together is a form of analysis called *content analysis*. You are identifying the broad concepts that respondents are referring to and noting their specific response. This is extremely time-consuming, takes a great deal of concentration and is really quite a sophisticated monitoring method to use. Detailed content analysis requires a great deal of skill and a great deal of care with its interpretation. I would not advocate this particular method of monitoring for the novice auditor. Steer clear of lengthy taped interviews for your early audits –

they should not be necessary, and while you are inexperienced in analysis they may not be terribly useful to you. As I have written before, there will be plenty of time to get to grips with more sophisticated techniques as you develop your knowledge and skills. I can understand the attraction of taping interviews with patients, and I can understand the wonderful richness of information that can be obtained. But some poor individual has to sit down and make real sense out of all that talk, and that is hard. Too hard for simple audits, in my opinion.

Taped interviews can be more useful if used for very structured interviews: interviews where you ask very plain questions which can be answered very simply, and are not ambiguous – questions that really can be answered 'Yes' or 'No'. In early audit, use the tape recorder only as a substitute for the pen – instead of giving patients questionnaires to fill in, ask them the questions and tape their yes, no or simple narrative response. Leave it at that.

For observation techniques you can use the same kind of grid principle as mentioned earlier. Again, take a large sheet of paper and draw a grid on it; across the top number each square as a number for your observations. So if you are going to observe the same intervention ten times, then you have ten squares numbered. Down the side you identify the criteria requiring the intervention to be observed. If you have turned your criteria into questions properly, then this should not give you a problem. For example, in the anaesthetic room standard there is a criterion that says the pre-theatre room is geared to children and that there are toys and books available. Our audit question then, needs to be 'Are there a range of toys and books available for children in the pre-theatre room?' You might want to audit this once a week for a month, making four observations in all. You would have four squares across the top and your audit question, or its code, at the side (see Figure 6.1 again).

If you want to use even less space, you can give your audit questions codes. I have already mentioned these codes a few times, and they are very simple. Coding can start very early on in the process with your standards. As you write each of the structure, process and outcome criteria, so you code them – S1, S2, P1, O1, and so on. (All of the standards in the figures are coded in this way.) Your audit questions then relate to these coded criteria, so when you write down your audit questions you also write next to them which code (for the criteria) that they refer to. When you come to draw up monitoring grids or summary sheets, you only need to use the code, rather than the whole audit question (see Figure 6.1). It is easy to do, easy to see and easy to make sense of.

You will now have one piece of paper with your standard on the front and your audit questions on the back. You have a second piece of paper (or you may need more) with your summary grid. These are the items you will use most and these are the items that you will need to keep. There will be back-up documentation of course – the original questionnaires from which you transferred information and other source documentation such as charts, care plans or patients' notes – but the information you will use most to make your conclusions and write your report will be the simple coded summary sheet, and the original standard.

Obviously, for those readers who have been involved in research projects none of this will be new – and in fact it may feel simplistic. But, as I have written previously, this book is aimed at nurses (and others) who have no prior knowledge of or skills in standard setting and monitoring and who need to be able to tackle audit in a systematic way without being afraid of the techniques.

If you have not been using summary sheets in your auditing, I think you will notice a big difference when you do start to use them. Groups that I have personally worked with have found them to be of significant benefit, particularly in helping them to feel less overwhelmed by the amount of data that has been collected. Well-collated and summarised data will make identifying the main findings of any monitoring exercise a much easier task.

The next step in the data-processing stage is to present your findings in a format that is simple to understand and can be shared with others. Depending on the size of your audit, this can be done as a simple written report, with the findings contained in the narrative. You may wish to use a table simply to list some of your information. If you are presenting your findings to people outside your immediate group, you may wish to make a more graphic, or pictorial presentation. In this case, you may wish to use a simple line graph or some sort of bar or pie chart.

Take, for example, a set of results from the anaesthetic room standard. The first thing to consider is how to define the groups of responses. Some of you may want to use percentages to describe your findings – for example, 75 per cent of parents said that they were satisfied with information given, 25 per cent expressed dissatisfaction. This sounds fine, until you come to consider that from a sample of twenty parents 75 per cent is only fifteen parents, and a 25 per cent dissatisfaction rate means that five parents were not happy. Percentages can be misleading – they can make your results appear to be representing a much larger number of people. This is not something that is usually deliberate (although it can be a mechanism for misleading one's audience), it is just that when per-centages are read from the page they give a sense of a large scale. When you read that 90 per cent of patients were satisfied you feel that this must be a very signifi-cant occurrence – but when you realise that 90 per cent means nine people out of a sample of ten and the de-partment sees 700 people per day (as might be the case in a large Out Patient Department) it is not quite so reassuring. So, if your sample size is small, do not automatically convert your figures into percentages. If you must, then qualify them in some way – try saying '90 per cent of patients (nine out of the ten sampled) were happy with the information'. Or simply 'Ten patients were sampled, of whom one expressed dissatisfaction (10 per cent)'.

The type of audit that is likely to be performed as a result of testing standards is probably going to use relatively small numbers. These can often be better presented in a graphic way. Bar charts are useful, accompanied by a brief explanation or, if you have quite a lot of information to present from the same question, then a pie chart may be helpful. Sometimes cartoons or a simple drawing can make a point far better than a lengthy explanation and a table.

Presenting results is important – it is the first stage in obtaining ownership of those results, and moving on to take action on them if this is necessary. If they are presented in a way that does not make sense to those listening or reading, or in a way that confuses them, then it is likely that the opportunity to do something positive will be lost, along with the interest and enthusiasm.

As with all presentations, not just those about audit, consider your audience and the purpose of the presentation. If you are presenting findings to the group which has been involved in the standard setting and monitoring, then it is quite likely that you will just need a simple narrative report that states the results or answers to each audit question and draws out the main areas of concern as simple conclusions. You may not need any table or diagram or graphics because it will be a small group and you can talk over the results together – clarifying as you go, referring back to the original data if necessary.

Perhaps your place of work has a regular seminar or study day where groups are invited to present their audit to colleagues; perhaps these meetings are multi-professional. In this situation, you are going to need to be a little more formal about your presentation. You may wish to use some graphic illustration such as simple bar charts to illustrate your findings. You could give these to the audience as a prepared handout or present them on an overhead projector – giving the results in figures orally and showing the distribution of results or comparison of results in a chart visually. This helps those present who know very little about your work, or what it entails to feel more involved in the process.

You may also find that following this kind of presentation to mixed or larger groups, people want to ask you questions about your methods, sample sizes and so on. It is wise to be prepared for this, and to be able to discuss why you need only small samples and why you have chosen to use particular methods. In multidisciplinary settings you may be challenged by someone who does not fully recognise the difference between research and audit and who takes you to task over your methods and the usefulness of your results. You should be prepared to answer these kinds of queries calmly and sensibly, making the points that were made earlier in the book – particularly those about requiring a quick feedback loop, and about not needing to generalise your results. It is better not to argue, just to explain that you seem to have a different understanding of audit, that is all.

There is always room for a little humour, particularly if you have assessed your audience well and know that it will be received positively. I recall one group who were quite creative in their presentation and used cartoons for a presentation of a simple audit that was being made to a large audience of audit novices. The audience was made up of nurses of varying nationality, with variable understanding of English. The audit was about the demographic and educational details of a small group from within the audience and had been undertaken as part of a small, participative group session. The sample was shown as ten matchstick people on an acetate, and results were overlaid on further acetates. For instance, the first set of results demonstrated the gender distribution in the sample – an overlaid acetate gave eight of the matchstick people skirts. The second set of results demonstrated the number with O or A level (or equivalent) qualifications and an overlaid acetate gave all of them scrolls in one hand. The third set of results demonstrated those with degrees, and an overlaid acetate gave five of them mortar boards – all of the males and three of the females. The presentation made the audience laugh, it made the results absolutely clear, and it certainly demonstrated that audit is not only about figures and tables. Remember though, do judge your audience and the appropriateness of your presentation – I can think of plenty of occasions when the above simple amusement would not have gone down very well!

There are also considerations of a more political nature when it comes to presenting results. Again, it is important to know your audience and how best they may be influenced. If your audience is largely nurses, you may wish to compare the results of their audit with similar audits from other wards or clinical areas – inject an element of competition and comparison. If your audience is made up of local managers, relate your findings to staffing levels, or educational needs or whatever may be appropriate. If you can find a financial or efficiency slant for an audience of managers that you are keen to influence, then this may be a very good way of doing it.

Before presenting your results to anyone, think hard about what your audience are going to be most interested in – what affects their working lives or the way that they operate and make decisions? Once you have a 'feel' for this, then build your presentation around these areas. You must relate your findings to your audience as much as you can. With a multidisciplinary audience this may mean that you have to vary your approach throughout the presentation, so that everyone can see what you are trying to achieve, or what you have done. A report which goes into a great deal of detail about the changes required in nursing practice will not hold the attention of managers. A report which tells them how changes may affect the efficiency of the service will. Be prepared to shift your emphasis to suit your listeners or readers. This advice holds good for any kind of presentation or written work and there are books and articles available that offer information that you can adapt for use with presenting your audit results. As with everything else associated with standard setting – the more of it you do, the better you will be at it.

At the end of this chapter you can:

● Identify different ways to present results
● Discuss the importance of knowing your audience.

CHAPTER 7

Getting Results (2)

Having completed your audit, the next step is to decide whether any action needs to be taken. Were your results as you expected? Was everything fine, or were there some areas where you did not comply with the criteria in the standard? Which areas did not comply, and was it by a large enough margin, or in an important enough area for you to need to do something about it? It is at this point that some people begin to consider 'weighting' their criteria. This means identifying those criteria that you think are most important, or at least, are more important than others. As you might expect, there is more than one school of thought about weighting criteria.

My own approach when working with groups is to encourage them to include only the essential 'business' in their standards. You will remember how previously, when considering criteria, it was suggested that you need to be very clear about what elements are absolutely relevant to the standard and to avoid getting 'hi-jacked' by related but not strictly relevant items. If you work like this and you consider that your criteria are all essential, then they are all equally important to fulfilling the standard, and there is no real need to weight them.

Others have a different view – some people argue that there will always be some criteria that are more important than others. For example, in our anaesthetic room standard, surely explaining things to parents is more important than having toys and books in the anaesthetic room? And some of you, I am sure will say 'Yes, it is'. It follows from this that if you fall down on the explanation criterion then you would take some action because it is an essential component; but if you fall down on the suitability of the environment then you may not take any action because it is not considered essential, or at least, not as important as some of the other criteria. If you want to work in this way, then do go on and allocate weightings to your criteria. It is best done at an earlier stage – probably when you have your final draft standard in front of you and you can consider all the criteria and decide on their relative importance. Do not forget that you will need the same agreement for your weightings that you needed for everything else. Everyone must be in the same mind about the priorities that are being set.

I have no problem with weighted criteria if you want to do that. It can encourage debating about what are the essential elements that make up good care. Such debate can only be good and useful. However, if you have followed the guidance on criteria writing from earlier on in the book then all your criteria are going to be relevant to achieving the standard. If they are not relevant then you will not have included them. I like to be very practical about these things, and it does seem to me to be wasted effort if you have criteria in your standard that you are going to ignore if you do not meet them. You may as well not include them in the first place. They are either all essential, or they do not need to be in the standard.

So, consider the pros and cons, and then make your own decision about weighting. Remember, there are no right or wrong ways of dealing with this – only different ways. If you think it is important to weight your criteria, then weight them. If you believe all your criteria are equally important for different reasons, then do not weight them. The important thing is that you understand why you have made your particular decision and what it means for your standard-setting programme in terms of the time and effort required.

Regardless of weighting issues, the point has been reached when recommendations need to be made based on the findings from your audit. Making plans to take action needs to be done as systematically as the rest of the process. When I first started standard setting, I did not consider action planning in the same way as writing the standard or preparing the audit tool. Once the standard had been audited, it was usually quite clear where things needed to be addressed and I would then leave it up to individual groups to go away and put things right. It soon became apparent that this kind of informal arrangement could be unreliable. Sometimes the necessary action was taken, but sometimes it was not and all the work that had been put into the standard would be wasted. It was at times such as this that I heard things like – 'Well, I knew this standard-setting business wouldn't work'. And 'All that paperwork for nothing, we won't bother again.'

If you want to avoid this, then you have to approach action planning formally and systematically. Look at your results. Which criteria have you not met? Make a list of them, and then put them in to some kind of priority order – which of them, as a group, do you feel need tackling immediately? At this point you may want to split them into two or three lists – problems that can be dealt with in the short term and those that might be more complex and need medium or longer-term approaches.

Once you have the problems listed, consider who can best deal with them. Are they nursing problems that you can deal with as a group? Does the root of the problem lie elsewhere? Is it out of your sphere of control? Will you need to bring in other professionals or workers to help solve the problem identified? In theory, this last difficulty ought not to arise. Think back again to the very beginning when you were first choosing a topic to write a standard about. At this very early stage you should have considered who needed to be involved, whether it was a purely nursing topic, or whether you would need others in your group. If you considered this carefully right at the start, then you should have the relevant people with you to enable you to take some remedial action. If you have not got those people, then you are going to have to bring in others very carefully indeed at this point. The whole agreement process will have to be gone through again, all the ownership work will have to be repeated. It is much better if you can make sure that the topic you are addressing is well within the sphere of control of your group members, and that you have the right group members to get the job done from the beginning.

Once you know which problems you are going to deal with first, and you have the relevant people available, then decide on the action that you need to take. This might seem obvious for some things, but for others you may have to think quite creatively about how to deal with the problem. The findings of the audit itself may offer some suggestions on what needs to be done. Think back to Chapter 6 when we considered the additional narrative material that may be offered in answer to simple questions – the response which suggested that information may not have been given in a completely appropriate way for lay people to understand. It is this kind of information from your audit that can be most helpful when it comes to thinking about your action plan.

There may be more than one approach to solving the problem, you may have to make a list of the options for action available to you and then agree upon the most appropriate. You may have certain constraints to take into consideration when you are planning your action. After all, there is not much point in making sure that your standards are achievable if the action you are planning to improve them is unrealistic. For example, do not decide that you need complicated teaching programmes if you have no access to anyone with the requisite knowledge. Do not decide that you need at least six extra trained staff to make a difference unless the person who holds your staffing budget has been a full and free participant in the whole process and is enthusiastically recognising the need.

Consider your options for action, consider the ones most likely to succeed, consider whether the action can all be done at once or if it would be better implemented in stages. Then make a choice about what you are going to do, and plan for that.

I have found that one of the most important elements of action planning is to decide *who* is going to be responsible for taking the action. You do need to have someone, or a number of people if necessary, who is clearly identified as being responsible for carrying out the required action. Allocating specific responsibilities is vital at this point. Some standards fail because although everyone agrees on the action that is required, no one bothers to do it, or everyone thinks that someone else is doing it. Named people who have accepted a clear responsibility for carrying out specific actions will ensure that something happens – particularly if you formalise your action plans on paper. It does not have to be elaborate, just unambiguous. Remember to put timescales to your required actions, (there is nothing like a deadline to motivate people) but, again, keep things realistic. A deadline is one thing, piling on the pressure is another. This is another one of those areas where your decisions may mean the difference between success and failure – requiring results too soon puts everyone under pressure, makes them feel resentful and may pre-determine failure. Too long a timescale and people lose interest, forget about it all and keep putting off the activity required on the grounds of having 'plenty of time to do this'.

Once you have agreed timescales for action to be taken, make sure everyone involved understands that after that time the action will be evaluated and the whole process will come back under review to assess progress and further action if necessary.

These elements will constitute a fairly formal action plan, and provide a checklist with which to evaluate the progress of the action plan. Unless action plans are documented, with clear responsibilities and realistic timescales, then work can sometimes peter out. Maintaining motivation and impetus in standard setting is a major task and should not be underestimated. Anything that helps the facilitator to do this should be utilised. Throughout the action-planning phase the group facilitator should be encouraging the group to set realistic goals and timescales, and should gently enquire about the progress of the action plan. A good facilitator will encourage the group to reflect on their action-planning activities – reminding them of particular learning points and emphasising lessons that will help them in the future. It is also important to give recognition and praise for what the group achieves and to encourage the group to explore the reasons why certain strategies may have failed, or been less successful than anticipated.

When groups are inexperienced, facilitators can help them to consider how they might present their results – including the success or failure of their action – in a way that makes the most impact and elicits the most support from others. Good facilitators will be continuously looking for opportunities to show how the standard-setting process helps people to take control of their own environment, make decisions that are based on good information and recognise the need to work as part of a team which is able to negotiate and agree.

Case Studies

The following three case studies briefly describe some of the projects I have been involved with. Their purpose is

76

to give you an idea of the kind of topics you can address using standard setting, and also the results possible to achieve.

Case 1

See Figure 2.2.

A long stay elderly care ward was known to have unacceptable levels of pressure sores. This was a long-standing problem and no one had really addressed it in the past. The staff were demoralised and demotivated, felt left out from mainstream hospital business, and felt that all their problems stemmed from being short of staff.

The facilitator could not just enter this situation and start standard setting. The staff of the ward were hostile and antagonistic. Initially the plan had to be one of winning the trust of the staff, and getting them to recognise that they had a problem and that they were the only people who could do anything about it. In this case the facilitator spent time visiting the ward, helping out, building up relationships. It took almost six months of regular weekly visits before the ward sister asked for help to deal with the problem – but this was a significant turning point. Without this particular ward sister's support, any action would have been pointless. Once recognition of the problem was obtained, then the facilitator suggested standard setting as a means of approaching the problem. This meant that the staff could not rush into looking for solutions but that they had to spend time thinking their way around the problem. By setting a standard which concentrated on providing care to meet patients' assessed needs, the group began, right at the beginning, to understand their responsibilities for care.

The criteria they identified included: using an assessment tool (and using it more than once!); documenting assessment and the care prescribed; developing a greater knowledge of current methods of preventing pressure damage, and so on. All went well – the standard was written and approved, the staff became more interested and excited about what they were doing, and the first monitoring exercise was planned. All this initial work had resulted in spectacularly improved care plans. Assessments were thorough and well documented, at risk scores were available and care was planned that reflected assessment. Excellent progress.

However, once monitoring began it soon became apparent that there was something wrong. Care planning was improved, documentation was exemplary – unfortunately when direct observation of care was undertaken and compared with care prescribed, there appeared to be some discrepancies. Practice had not yet changed – everyone was diligently writing down what they were supposed to do, but were not doing it – they were still using the same methods as previously and were still operating in the same old way. This was immediately apparent from the monitoring and therefore could be addressed. The documentation checks did show all was well – and had the auditor not double checked with some direct observation of care the problem might have remained unresolved for a little while longer.

A second phase of work was planned which concentrated on patients receiving care identified in the care plan. A specific criterion was included in the standard to reflect this – so that everyone knew exactly what they were expected to do. This work took almost two years to complete in total. By the end of the two-year period, pressure damage had been reduced to below national average levels, the staff had begun to take a renewed interest in their work, and had started to write more standards addressing different issues which they had identified for themselves. Not only did this simple standard improve things for the patients, but it also encouraged significant changes in the attitude of the staff on the ward.

Two years later these previously demotivated and demoralised people were using team nursing, were planning a trial of primary nursing, gave talks to other groups of staff who were starting out on standard setting, and had many visitors to their ward as a demonstration site for change through participation in monitoring practice. They had learned how to take control of their own situation. Standard setting had been a means of empowering them.

For the facilitator, change here, though hard won, meant that the possibilities for change in other, more receptive places, could be limitless. There was a huge sense of achievement.

Case 2

See Figure 7.1.

A group of theatre staff wanted to improve the preparation of patients for theatre – not their physical preparation but their emotional readiness: for example, the level of information given to them. They approached the facilitator with a fairly clear idea of what they wanted to do and a great deal of enthusiasm about getting started. The facilitator encouraged them to slow down a little and consider the ward staff. She raised the following issues: who is responsible for preparing patients for theatre? In which location is the patient's prime carer likely to be? The ward staff undoubtedly felt it was theirs, and also felt that they did it reasonably well. The theatre staff, by virtue of the fact that they wanted to do something different, were threatening the ward staff, whether they intended to or not. They wanted to go to the wards, talk to patients who were going to theatre and give them information about what was to happen to them.

The first stage was to consider whether there was any ward in the hospital that was open to what the theatre staff were proposing and which might be willing to act as a trial area. One particular specialist area agreed to

Figure 7.1
Standard Setting Text

STANDARD STATEMENT: ALL PATIENTS FOR ELECTIVE SURGERY RECEIVE A PRE-OPERATIVE VISIT FROM A THEATRE NURSE		
STRUCTURE	PROCESS	OUTCOME
S1 A trained nurse is available for routine ward visits between 1400 and 2000 hours Sunday–Thursday.	P1 The theatre nurse approaches the patient in a calm, informal and reassuring manner.	01 The patient states that the pre-operative visit was helpful to them.
S2 All theatre nurses are aware of the possible anxieties that the patients and/or their relatives may have associated with going to theatre.	P2 In discussion with the patient and/or his or her relatives, the theatre nurse highlights likely events, and encourages the patient to ask any questions he or she may have about his or her visit to theatre.	02 Theatre and ward staff feel that pre-operative visits contribute to the continuity of patient care.
S3 An agreed philosophy for pre-operative visiting is available in theatre and on surgical wards.	P3 The theatre nurse ensures that the ward staff are aware of his or her presence on the ward, that any relevant information or request is passed on to appropriate ward or theatre staff and documented in nursing notes.	
S4 Photographs and general printed information relating to theatre are available.	P4 If patients request it, pre-operative visits can be arranged to coincide with visiting hours.	

join the theatre staff in the project. The standard they wrote was about increasing patients' awareness of what to expect when they go to theatre. In collaboration with ward staff it was agreed that a designated member of theatre staff would be available between certain times to talk to patients on the ward booked for surgery on the following day. This person would not wear theatre greens but would wear ward uniform, and would have with her a set of photographs of the theatre area which showed

80

members of staff in theatre uniform, gowned and masked, and also the anaesthetic room and the theatre itself. The order of events would be explained and talked through and the patients encouraged to ask any questions that they might have. The theatre nurse would also arrange to talk to patients with their relatives if this was what they wanted.

The standard was written and approved with the ward staff. By working through the standard together a number of potential problems were avoided. For example, the ward staff felt it was important that the theatre staff did not just appear on the ward without any warning in case it disrupted usual patterns of care, or plans that were in place for the patient. It was agreed right from the start that theatre staff would inform the ward staff of their availability and would report to the nurse in charge when they arrived on the ward to let her know who they wanted to see, to check it was convenient. This saved wasted journeys to the ward, and disappointed patients not getting the visits they were expecting. Communication between the ward staff and theatre staff improved and a greater sense of a team approach to caring for patients undergoing surgery was developed. As a result of its initial success, the scheme was extended to other ward areas and became a part of normal practice.

The facilitator, having made sure that everyone who needed to be involved was involved, could just sit back and let this one happen. The initial enthusiasm was there, the idea was good, and relatively well developed before the project started. The only real input needed was in constructing the monitoring tool and advising on the audit.

Case 3

See Figures 7.2 and 7.3.

The two previous studies have been about tackling problems, specifically improving care in a particular way.

81

Figure 7.2
Standard Setting Text

Standard Statement: All patients requiring social care on discharge have their needs assessed, an individual plan made, and are discharged in a timely manner into an environment suitable for their needs.

STRUCTURE	PROCESS	OUTCOME
S1 Social Care team (SCT) consists of: 1 on site manager, 4.5 qualified social workers,1 social work asst.	P1 Patients admitted electively will be assessed for social care need at pre-admission clinic and this assessment documented in discharge plan within the nursing notes.	O1 Patients requiring social care on discharge are identified as soon as possible after admission.
S2 Office accomodation and access to facilities for 1.5 WTE secretarial staff for the SCT are provided by the host Trust.	P2 If the patient is an emergency/arranged admission the nurse with prime responsibility for the patient's care will assess his or her need for social care as soon after admission as possible and document this in the nursing notes.	O2 The patient and his/her carer state that they felt involved in the social care planning process.
S3 The SCT is available between the hours of 9:00am and 5:00pm, Monday to Thursday and 9:00am to 4:00pm Friday.	P3 The nurse makes any necessary referral to the SCT within 24 hours of the patient's admission to the ward by discharge planning form.	O3 The patient is discharged into the most appropriate environment of their choice and with the relevant services arranged to meet their needs.
S4 Out of hours emergency cover for problems other than discharge planning is provided by Emergency Duty Team.	P4 Where the need for social care on discharge is not apparent on admission, the nurse with prime responsibility for the patient's care refers to the SCT as soon as she/he becomes aware of a possible need.	O4 Hospital staff and Social Care staff feel that communication is enhanced and working relationships improved.
	P5 The SCT acknowledges receipt of referrals within 24 hours (1 working day) following receipt of referral.	O5 The patient and his/her carer state that they were informed of services available and their likely eligibility.
S5 The SCT give three weeks' notice in writing to the appropriate Ward Managers of any planned temporary break in service.	P6 The SCT respond to the referral within 48 hours (2 working days).	
S6 Relevant discharge/social care planning documentation is available on each ward.	P7 Where above response is not possible, SCT documents reasons in nursing notes.	
	P8 The SCT assesses the patient in collaboration with the responsible nurse, other relevant professionals, the patient and his/her carer using the criteria specified by the SCT.	
S7 All ward nursing staff and other relevant professionals are aware of the criteria for referral to the SCT and the means of making the referral.	P9 The SCT details services required and requested and agrees this with health care team, the patient and his/her carer. This is documented in nursing notes.	
	P10 The SCT give the patient, in writing, a named contact with telephone number for follow up of community social services.	

Figure 7.3
Standard Setting Text

Method	Code	Audit Question
Observe	S1	Are Social Services maintaining full establishment?
Observe	S2	Are agreed office accommodation, facilities and secretarial staff provided?
Check all wards	S6	Is relevant discharge/social care documentation available?
Check nursing documents and SCT documents	P2	Are emergency patients assessed for social care needs as soon as possible after admission (judgement)?
Check nursing documents and discharge planning form.	P3	Is the discharge planning form (DPF) completed and sent to the SCT Dept within 24 hours of admission?
Check nursing documents and DPF	P4	If referral is late, is reason documented?
Check nursing documents	P5	Are acknowledgement slips attached to relevant nursing documents?
Check nursing documents	P6	Has the SCT responded within 48 hours of referral?
Check nursing documents	P9	Are services required and services agreed documented by SCT member?
Ask nurses and ward clerks	S3	Are you always able to contact SCT within working hours?
Ask nurses	S4	Can each nurse state who he/she would contact for out-of-hours social care support?
Ask nurses	S5	When the SCT Department has been closed (e.g Xmas) did you receive adequate notice?
Ask selection of professionals	S7	Can each person state the relevant criteria for referral to SCT?
Ask selection of professionals	P8	Does each person feel that there has been collaboration between professionals and relatives in assessment of SCT need?
Ask selection of professionals	O4	Does each person feel that relationships and communication have improved since SLA was introduced?
Ask patients	P10	Were you given a contact name and number to ring in case services did not turn up?
Ask patients	02	Were you involved in the plans for your discharge?
Ask patients	04	Were you told which services you were eligible for?
Ask patients	03	Were the services arranged adequate?

Standards can also be used for other purposes. For instance they can be used as a clarifying mechanism in order to make difficult tasks a little easier.

Case 3 is a multidisciplinary project involving nursing staff and Social Services. The Social Services team had agreed a service level agreement with the management of the hospital. This agreement was quite straightforward, and was formally written as a description of services agreed, covering some three or four A4 pages. The social care team wanted to monitor the service level agreement to see how they were shaping up, but did not know where to start.

The facilitator in this instance suggested that the first step might be to draw out some of the sentences in the service level agreement that could be identified as targets or standards that they needed to meet. After working through the document a number of sentences were identified and written down separately – these included items such as:

- the number of support staff that the hospital had agreed to provide

- the timescales that the social care team had agreed to work within

- the specific activities that had been agreed between both parties.

From this it was easy to see how these sentences might become criteria within a standard by working on them a little. They had to be sorted into structure, process and outcome but with a little thought this was not too difficult to achieve. Figure 7.2 shows the resulting standard.

The criteria involving nursing staff were naturally negotiated with the relevant staff, and the standard finally agreed. This part of the work took most time, as the people involved from Social Services had no previous experience of writing standards and had not come across structure, process, outcome before. However, they quickly picked up what was required and within three meetings a standard was refined and ready for wider approval. Two, hour-long, meetings later a monitoring tool had been developed. Within three months, the team had gone from having a wordy service level agreement that was detailed and difficult to measure, to having two sheets of paper which made explicit everyone's responsibilities within the agreement, and a simple monitoring tool which could be used at any time they felt ready. Figures 7.2 and 7.3 illustrate both the standard and the monitoring tool.

Even though this book has been written primarily for nurses, I am sure that it is easy to see how standard setting can be used by anyone, to deal with a range of issues. You do not have to be a nurse, and it does not have to address purely issues of clinical care or professional practice. This last case illustrates how standards solved an administrative difficulty, how to monitor a contract or agreement in a sensible and simple manner. This is my most recent experience of success with standards, and it has certainly encouraged me to carry on using the method to help with non-clinical issues as well as aspects of care.

At the end of this chapter you will have considered:

- Issues concerning the weighting of criteria

- The role of action planning

- A range of situations where standard setting can be useful.

CHAPTER 8

Encouraging Change

Up to this chapter, this book has dealt with the 'mechanics' of standard setting – how to write a standard that means something to you; how to construct a simple monitoring tool that is relevant to the standard that you have written; how to collect the data that you need; and how to put together an action plan for improving the activity related to your standard. I hope it has been practical and clear and that you feel confident enough to try out the process for yourself. If you have been putting the guidance in the book into practice as you have read it, then I hope that you are pleased with the finished result. With practice it will get easier, you will be able to write standards and prepare monitoring tools quickly, and it will integrate naturally into your working practice.

The mechanics of standard setting are not as easy as they look, but neither are they as complicated as you may sometimes be led to believe. Mastering the mechanics, however, is only the beginning. Being able to produce standards and measuring tools and action plans is only a small part of the story. At the end of the day, what really matters is the *difference* you are able to make to care, to the patient's experience, to your own practice, to your colleagues' attitudes. Making this difference is about putting your action plans into practice – it is about bringing about change.

There are very many books and articles to be read on

change and change management. I do not suppose that I am going to add anything new to what has already been written by people far more experienced than I am. The remainder of this book will remind you of how change comes about and how hard you have to work at it to make it really happen. At the end you will see how standards are themselves a mechanism for change and with the right facilitation and careful implementation they will do much more for you than identify guidelines for good practice.

Change does not just happen. It is engineered, it is caused by someone or something, and for it to be a positive rather than a negative experience it needs to be a managed process – and a well-managed process. At the time of writing it is probably safe to say that most people reading this book will be feeling punch drunk with change; Government reforms, organisational upheavals, education swings and roundabouts, shifting priorities, remodelling, reprofiling, re-engineering, reshaping. Whatever we call it, it is still change, and it is not always well managed – if it was we might not feel quite so cynical or so apprehensive about it all. Our own experiences, generally speaking, should serve to ensure that we, whenever we have an opportunity to bring about change, do it with care and consideration.

Most readers of this book will be able to tell a story which illustrates how change can be mismanaged. We can think of large scale mismanagement of change – at the beginning of the book we considered the introduction of the 'nursing process', where nurses all over the country repeated the same mistakes and suffered the long-term consequences (and are still suffering them now in some places nearly twenty years later). Smaller, more local difficulties also come to mind. I can think of my own personal disasters – failing to involve key people; using previously successful strategies that proved to be inappropriate in a new situation; mostly just trying to move too quickly. This last point is fundamental in change management – it is a process which takes a long time – much longer than you might expect. No matter how long you have been working as a change agent, or how many successful projects you have under your belt, you still want to move more quickly than you should with the latest one. 'Take your time' can be a particularly painful lesson to learn, but a very necessary one.

Consider some of the experiences you have of the change process – think particularly about processes that were not very successful or straightforward. Were there any common factors? How much time was spent in preparing for the proposed change? How much time was spent on the implementation of the change? None at all? Just a week or two? How much discussion was there? How much agreement? Time is a factor in all change processes that you can not afford to skimp on. Change takes as long as it takes.

People perceive the prospect of change in different ways. To some it will be an exciting opportunity to try something fresh, to clear out old ways and practices, to make a new start. To others it will disturb their carefully nurtured status quo, throw up the unexpected and create turmoil where there was pleasant equilibrium. There are those who find change of any kind anxiety provoking and fearsome – will they be able to cope with new circumstances, new ways? Will they like what happens around them, or to them? Still others find the possibility of change very threatening – will they have to give up, or lose control over things? Will they be expected to act in ways that they have never had to act before? Will different skills be required of them? Quite often people are afraid of what the change might mean for them. Will it expose their lack of knowledge or confidence? Will they look foolish while learning new skills, will someone else take over their position in the hierarchy because they already have the new skills? All these reasons will affect how people respond to proposed changes.

Some people respond negatively for very basic reasons – they dislike the person who is proposing the change or acting as the spokesperson. Personality clashes have brought many excellent projects shuddering to a halt and can be particularly difficult to deal with. Some people respond negatively to change not because they think it is a bad idea, or because they disagree in principle – their negative response may come from the fact that they did not think of the idea themselves, or that they really want to lead the change process themselves but for some reason are unable to. Professional jealousy can also be a killer of innovation. If you have had a number of successes, always be aware that there may be someone who is just waiting for you to fall flat on your face – who may be willing even to help you to fall flat on your face. It sounds petty and nasty, but it happens; and it can happen at all levels of organisations.

Being a change agent is not always about excitement and satisfaction, it can also be quite a painful experience, and sometimes you do have to give up and leave things alone. Try to be as well prepared as possible – know the culture of your organisation and the people you are working with, find out who is going to be with you from the beginning, try not to antagonise anyone, and keep explaining and encouraging active involvement. If it does get tough, remind yourself that you knew that it was not going to be easy, and that it will be worth it in the long term. Understand why people respond to the prospect of change in different ways and try to work out strategies for dealing with them.

Never underestimate the importance of getting as many people as possible on your side – for your own support, as well as for maintaining momentum. It is also useful to make contact with other people who are working as change agents so that experiences can be shared and peer support can be obtained. There are formal networks for this – the King's Fund Nursing Development Network is one and the Royal College of Nursing Quality Assurance Network (QUAN) another – or you might set up a support network for people working in similar ways in your local area, or in your own organisation.

You can increase your chances of having a positive reaction to proposed change. There are some key principles to work through. Many of you reading this will have come across the three phases of change, identified as 'unfreezing', 'changing' and 'refreezing' by Kurt Lewin in the 1950s. This is a simple model to remember, and those three words act as reminders of the activities you will need to work through.

Unfreezing is about loosening up the way that people think about the current situation, helping them to recognise a need to change. It means helping them to see that there are other options available to them, that there are other approaches, that the current way is not the only way. Unfreezing can take a while. This is the stage where you employ all the help that you can – by providing as much information as possible. If a group thinks that standard setting might be a useful way forward for them, then find them articles (books even!), enlist people who have been successful with the technique to come and talk to them, show them examples from other clinical areas or hospitals. Do not push them, give them time to assimilate the information and make a reasoned choice. If you can get an opinion leader to feel positive about it, perhaps the ward sister or nurse specialist or practice development nurse, then they will influence the stragglers or the undecided. Whatever it is that you want to change, whether it is introducing standard setting or implementing your action plan at the end of the standard-setting process, you need to provide as much information and give people as much preparation as possible. Talk about alternative methods, get people involved in presenting small seminars or talks, use anything you can to encourage exploration of alternatives.

During the standard-setting process let people decide for themselves what it needs to be about. Provide education – if there are new skills needed in order to effect the change, let the group decide what they are and the best way of providing them. If you need to provide education and training, remember to go at a pace which suits everyone – let your enthusiasts move ahead when they are ready, but continue to provide the education and training for the slower participants. All those who will be affected by the change need to be *involved* in the planning and implementation of it – participation is the key word. Participation helps to develop ownership and ownership helps to develop a responsibility for making it work out.

All of these are elements of unfreezing, and the unfreezing process never really stops; it merges imperceptibly into the 'changing' phase. If you try to move into changing without doing any unfreezing, then I think you will find it quite a difficult process. Probably all of my bad experiences of change have been as a result of insufficient attention being paid to the unfreezing, preparation stage. It can not be bypassed.

For example, one of the most successful projects I have worked on was the standard outlined in Case 1 in Chapter 7. A group of nurses needed to tackle the incidence of pressure damage on their ward. The biggest problem facing me as their facilitator was the fact that they did not recognise the problem. Pressure sore incidence had been identified in a survey, and their ward had come out fairly badly. In spite of this, there was no motivation to do anything differently. Their view was that the problem was all caused by things that were outside of their control – not enough staff, too many unqualified staff, inadequate equipment, and so on. They were unable to see the real reasons – outdated working methods, lack of education and expertise, inability to apply theory to practice.

Somehow, these feelings had to be altered before any alteration of practice was likely to take place. Initial facilitation was not about alternative ways of working but about changing their attitudes. A great deal of time had to be spent building up relationships – just visiting the ward, chatting to the staff about the day-to-day difficulties, gaining acceptance as someone who could help with other things, not just the pressure sore problem. The first issue in the unfreezing stage was to get the staff to see their facilitator as a supportive helper – not someone sent in by managers to 'sort them out'.

Once a level of trust had been built up, the second stage could begin: a re-educative phase where methods of preventing pressure damage could be revisited without the group feeling patronised or stupid. Different ways of organising their workload could be discussed as a means of using existing staff more efficiently, and of sharing the work more fairly. No changes could have been brought about without going through this. Setting a standard became a part of this stage, some time into the actual change process. The group had to sit down and decide what it was they needed to have, and needed to do, in order to improve their incidence of pressure damage. Writing criteria for a standard was an excellent way of refining these views and prioritising their need for action. Planning care more systematically was one area identified, and making better use of risk assessment tools. Increasing their expertise in prevention methods was another, along with making better use of the equipment and aids available to them. Writing the standard helped them to feel in control of what was happening, and to plan any changes at their own pace and to fit their own constraints.

Implementing the standard and actually making the changes was relatively easy as a result of all the groundwork. Moving away from task allocation was frustrating but ultimately rewarding. Team nursing, though planned and carefully implemented, did not work straight away.

There were pockets of resistance which meant that delaying the project was a real possibility. Determination won the day, however – the need for change was recognised as more important than keeping the peace, and stragglers were enthusiastically encouraged by their colleagues. Working patterns were changed, prevention methods were brought up to date and practised by everyone, resources were better utilised. Pressure sore incidence reduced dramatically. Throughout this period the facilitator was around – supporting, providing information, encouraging others to take the lead and to make decisions. The ward become a model for others who were trying to use standard setting, self-esteem went up, confidence went up and all things considered, the exercise was a complete success.

The refreezing process was enhanced by the levels of success achieved. Because there was wide recognition throughout the organisation of the amount of change that had been achieved, and of the efforts put in to bring it about, the group of nurses felt valued for their achievement, were proud of the changes they had made and of the measurable improvements to care that they could demonstrate. There was no way that they would let things slip! The cycle for them was complete. New behaviours were 'frozen' into place.

Refreezing, however, does not always occur. A lot depends upon the level of commitment to the work in the first place, and how worthwhile the results appear to be. Often there is a temporary freeze followed by a thaw and a return to old, well-established ways. Making sure that changes last is one of the most difficult elements of the process. For a facilitator it means continuing to be around, to offer encouragement, to praise, to check back, to emphasise with groups that efforts have been worthwhile and continue to be so. For a facilitator, the cycle never ends.

Standard setting is not an end product – it is a means

to an end. For the group in the preceding example, writing the standard was not their aim, but it helped them to achieve their aim. In fact, it helped them to achieve a number of aims, some of which were only identified through the standard-writing process. The example quoted is also a good example of how standard setting does not stand alone. It is a part of an educative, problem-solving process which can help build confidence and encourage action. The facilitator is a crucial element – poor facilitation may mean nothing happens, or that groups are antagonised and fail to see, or use, the possible benefits. A good facilitator will leave behind a revitalised group, motivated to continue and confident of further success.

In Case 3 in Chapter 7, the members of the social care team involved in writing the standard were amazed at how much they had been able to achieve and how far they had moved from a situation of not knowing where to begin to having a clear way forward planned out in front of them. They now want to use their new-found skills in other areas of their work. Having discovered one significant benefit, they are keen to use it to realise others.

Standard setting on its own does not change practice significantly, but joined together with education, motivation, and support it is a tool that has incredible potential for making a real difference. The standard setting cycle as described by the Royal College of Nursing below, can be fitted easily into a connected series of three much wider concepts, all of which have an increasing emphasis in

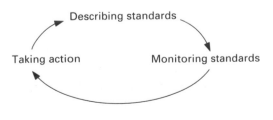

Describing standards

Taking action   Monitoring standards

the future of nursing. If you have understood the connecting activity in the standard-setting cycle, then it will be a small step to seeing how this fits into a much bigger picture.

Describing care becomes the concept of identifying standards and indicators for any aspect of the service, monitoring becomes audit (whether professional or organisational) and taking action becomes service development. We now have a much bigger cycle to make our way around, and a cycle which can affect every element of the work that we do.

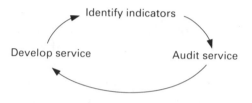

This might be the quality assurance cycle, it might be the audit cycle, it might be a grander version of the standard-setting cycle, it might be the change cycle. I am sure that you will have seen something similar described in all of these terms. For me it is simply a means of going forward – it is the wheel which propels us into the future in a systematic and logical way, one stage at a time, and at our own pace. We can control this cycle – but first we have to get on to it.

In Chapter 7 I provided three examples of how standard setting had helped in three different situations. I could provide any number of others; for example, how the meals service for elderly patients was improved, increasing the opportunities for clients to choose their own food regardless of their sensory disability; how the level of safety in a childrens' play area was improved, using the expertise of nursery nurses and resulting in staff taking greater responsibility, and feeling in control of their

Figure 8.1
Standard Setting Text

STANDARD STATEMENT: ALL VERBAL AND WRITTEN INFORMATION REGARDING INFANTS AND THEIR FAMILIES REMAINS CONFIDENTIAL		
STRUCTURE	PROCESS	OUTCOME

S1 All nursing staff are aware of their responsibilities in ensuring and maintaining confidentiality of information regarding infants and their families.
 	
S2 All nursing staff have access to:
  i) Standard of care
  ii) Guidelines for clinical practice
  iii) Grievance and disciplinary procedures
  iv) UKCC advisory paper on confidentiality (clause 9)
  v) Code of Professional Conduct
 	
S3 A notes trolley and folders to hold medical records and nursing notes are available on the Unit.
 	
S4 Experienced trained staff are available to give handover reports.
 	
S5 A telephone is available away from the nursing station for liaison calls with community services and other departments to be taken in privacy
	P1 The nurse in charge ensures that the handover is not overheard by anyone other than staff involved.
	
	P2 Nursing staff do not discuss the infants' condition with visitors, but refer enquiries to the parents for information.
	
	P3 Nursing staff ensure that telephone conversations are not overheard.
	
	P4 Nursing staff discourage visitors and parents from viewing other babies' charts.
	
	P5 Nursing staff ensure that parents and visitors are restricted to the nursery of their baby only.
	
	P6 Nursing staff ensure that all visitors wait in waiting rooms while the ward round is in progress.
	
	P7 Parents may remain on the Unit while their own baby is under discussion; but must leave when other babies are being discussed.
		O1 Verbal handover report is given in privacy and in strictest confidence.
		
		O2 No information is given to visitors or unauthorised persons without the consent of the parents.
		
		O3 Written medical and nursing reports are not accessible to unauthorised persons.
		
		O4 All information regarding infants and their families remains confidential.

own workplace; improving the level of confidentiality in a special care baby unit without having to restrict the movement or activities of parents and relatives. Some of these standards, and examples of others, are included as Figures 8.1, 8.2 and 8.3 of this book or are referred to in the 'Further Reading'. They all represent real changes being made, and real improvements resulting from them. But, in spite of all this, there are no rules and regulations for success. At the end of the day it will depend on the nature of the problem, the way it is approached, and the context of the situation. I also believe, and this is purely

Figure 8.2
Standard Setting Text

STANDARD STATEMENT: ALL PLAY TAKES PLACE IN A SAFE ENVIRONMENT		
STRUCTURE	PROCESS	OUTCOME
S1 There is a Nursery Nurse on duty between 7:30am and 7:00pm every day.	P1 The Nursery Nurse ensures that the play area is supervised at all times.	O1 Children do not come to any harm as a result of faulty or unsuitable toys in the playroom.
S2 Both play areas are stocked with play materials/toys suitable for children aged 0–8 years, with specific regard to their safety.	P2 The Nursery Nurse checks all donated toys and equipment for their safety and suitability for use with children aged 0–8 years.	O2 A safe environment is maintained.
S3 The Nursery Nurse has knowledge of safety aspects to be considered in the playroom.	P3 The Nursery Nurse constantly observes the play area and play materials/toys for safety hazards.	
S4 The Nursery Nurse is aware of the procedure for reporting faulty equipment.	P4 The Nursery Nurse advises parents on the suitability of toys to be brought into the ward.	

an opinion, that the personal qualities of the facilitator have a great deal to do with it. Change theory can be learned, skills can be practised, but at the end of the day, a patient and helping person is required. I have met facilitators who have had all of the skills and knowledge to bring about change but none of the personal attributes, and have failed miserably. I have met others who have the right kind of personality and none of the 'formal' training or theory who still manage to get things done by taking their colleagues along with them. I think that quite a lot of people will probably disagree with me, but I think there is such a thing as a 'natural' facilitator, and that these people have the most success in terms of bringing about lasting change and enhancing the experience of their colleagues. If you find one, make the most of him or her, tell your manager about this person's skills and how he or she could be more widely used in the organisation!

Figure 8.3
Standard Setting Text

STANDARD STATEMENT. PATIENTS WISHING TO SELF-ADMINISTER PRESCRIBED MEDICATION ARE ASSESSED AND GIVEN RELEVANT INFORMATION PRIOR TO COMMENCING SELF-MEDICATION PROGRAMME		
S1 Qualified nurses have knowledge of the self-medication programme.	P1 A qualified nurse assesses the patient to determine his or her capabilities to participate in the programme using the approved assessment form.	O1 Patients who are assessed as suitable for the programme are able to tell the nurse and the pharmacist about the dosage, actions and side effects of their medication prior to participating in the programme.
S2 Qualified nurses have knowledge of the patient's medication including dosage, actions and side effects.	P2 The nurse explains the programme to the patient and gives literature to reinforce the information given. The nurse offers opportunities for the patient to question and discuss the programme.	O2 Patients who are assessed as suitable for the programme are aware of the self-medication programme and its implications.
S3 Literature explaining the self-medication programme is available on the ward.	P3 The patient, nurse and doctor sign the approved form giving consent for inclusion in the programme.	
S4 Time is set aside for nurses to assess patients and inform them of programme.	P4 The nurse informs the pharmacist of the patients who are able to participate in the programme.	
S5 Medical staff are aware of the self-medication programme.	P5 The pharmacist and nurse explain the patient's medication (see assessment checklist).	
S6 A pharmacist is available for patient education concerning self-medication.	P6 The nurse documents that the self-medication assessment criteria have been followed.	

CHAPTER 9

Have Framework . . . Will Succeed?

Having a mechanism to work through when trying to bring about change is extremely useful. I have found this particular framework of setting and monitoring standards to be successful and rewarding. But a framework on its own cannot make changes – success is dependent upon taking on board the whole philosophy of participation, education, involvement and facilitation as well as the mechanics. It also helps to have a high level of personal commitment, a vision of what might be achieved, and a clear understanding that in order to change practice one needs to change people – that is the most challenging aspect of all. In order to bring about change you have to believe that change is possible – and you have to be able to make others believe that change is possible too. Being able to offer practical ways of tackling changes is a useful skill to have.

With this book in your pocket, and an unswerving belief that things can and should be different, you should be able to make a start in your work area on setting local standards and monitoring them, taking remedial action and building positive and enthusiastic teams for taking work forward. Good luck!

Further Reading

Standard setting

Baker, C. and Girvin, J. (1991) Standard setting in paediatrics. *Nursing Standard*, 5(25): 32–4.

Dunn, C. (1990) Improving intensive care. *Nursing Times*, 86(12): 32–4.

Evans, K. and Corrigan, P. (1992) Standard setting: an introduction to differing approaches. *Nursing Practice*, 4(3): 16–19.

Girvin, J. (1990) Standard setting in paediatrics. *Nursing*, 4(13): 26–8.

Girvin, J. (1990) Standard setting in practice. *Nursing*, 4(12): 11–13.

Girvin, J. (1990) Setting standards – uphill work. *Nursing Standard*, 4(44): 35.

Girvin, J. (1991) Deals on meals. *Nursing Times*, 87(34): 38–40.

Lang, N. and Wessel Krejci, J. (1991) Standards and holism: a reframing. *Holistic Nursing Practice*, 5(3): 14–21.

Royal College of Nursing (1990) *Quality Patient Care: The Dynamic Standard Setting System*, Scutari, London.

Royal College of Nursing. *Standards of Care* series. Scutari, London.

Tingle, L. (1992) Legal implications of standard setting in nursing. *British Journal of Nursing*, 1(14): 728–31.

Related interest

Andrews, M. (1993) Importance of nursing leadership in implementing change. *British Journal of Nursing.* 2(8): 437–9.

Bond, S. and Thomas, L. (1991) Issues in measuring outcomes of nursing. *Journal of Advanced Nursing.* 16: 1492–1502.

Davidhizar, R. (1993) Leading with charisma. *Journal of Advanced Nursing*, 18: 675–9.

Donabedian, A. (1981) Advantages and limitations of explicit criteria for assessing the quality of health care. *Millbank Memorial Quarterly/Health and Society.* 59(1): 99–106.

Heron, J. (1989) *The Facilitators Handbook.* London, Kogan Page.

Irvine, D. and Irvine, S. (eds) (1991) *Making Sense of Audit.* Oxford, Radcliffe Medical Press.

Kitson, A. and Harvey, G. (1991) *A Bibliography of Nursing Quality Assurance and Standards 1932–1987.* London, Scutari Press.

Lewin, K. (1946) Action research and minority problems. *Journal of Social Issues*, 2: 34–46.

Redfern, S. and Norman, I. (1990) Measuring the quality of nursing care: a consideration of differing approaches. *Journal of Advanced Nursing*, 15: 1260–71.

Salvage, J. (1990) So you want to do audit. . . . *Nursing Standard.* 5(3): 53–4.

Schiber, S. and Larson, E. (1991) Evaluating the quality of caring: structure, process and outcome. *Holistic Nursing Practice.* 5(3): 57–66.

Wright, C. and Whittington, D. (1992) *Quality Assurance – an Introduction for Health Care Professionals.* Churchill Livingstone, London.

Further information about the Dynamic Standard Setting System (DySSSy) can be obtained from:

RCN Dynamic Quality Improvement programme
National Institute for Nursing
Radcliffe Infirmary
Woodstock Road
Oxford OX2 6HE

DySSSy can now be implemented with the support of a piece of software called the DQI Toolbox. Information on this software is also available at the above address.

The RCN DQI programme runs a network for nurses and others interested in improving quality of care, and for those using DySSSy as a prime method. This is the DQI network (which replaces the QUAN network) and further information is available again from the DQI programme in Oxford.

Index